STRUCTURED CLINICAL INTERVIEW FOR DSM-IV AXIS I DISORDERS

SCID-I

CLINICIAN VERSION

Administration Booklet

Michael B. First, M.D.
Robert L. Spitzer, M.D.
Miriam Gibbon, M.S.W.
Janet B. W. Williams, D.S.W.

Biometrics Research Department
New York State Psychiatric Institute
Department of Psychiatry
Columbia University
New York, New York

Please visit www.scid4.org for more information about the SCID

Manufactured in the United States of America on acid-free paper
15 14 13 12 4 3 2 1

American Psychiatric Publishing, A Division of American Psychiatric Association
1000 Wilson Boulevard
Arlington, VA 22209-3901
www.appi.org

ISBN 978-1-58562-453-9

For citation: First MB, Spitzer RL, Gibbon M, Williams JBW: Structured Clinical Interview for DSM-IV Axis I Disorders—Clinician Version (SCID-CV). Washington, DC, American Psychiatric Press, 1997. Copyright © 1997 Michael B. First, Robert L. Spitzer, Miriam Gibbon, and Janet B. W. Williams.

Available From American Psychiatric Publishing:

Structured Clinical Interview for DSM-IV Axis I Disorders (SCID-I)—Clinician Version,

- User's Guide (order #8931)
  The User's Guide contains detailed instructions for administering the SCID, guiding you through the interview process and demonstrating how to make accurate DSM-IV diagnoses.
- Administration Booklet (order #8932)
  The spiral-bound, reusable Administration Booklet contains the interview questions and the DSM-IV diagnostic criteria.
- Packet of five Scoresheets (order #8933)
  One-time-use Scoresheets contain the abridged DSM-IV diagnostic criteria and provide space for recording diagnostic decisions and descriptive information.
- Administration Booklet + packet of five Scoresheets (order #8934)
- User's Guide + Administration Booklet + packet of five Scoresheets (order #8935)

The **Research Version** of the SCID is available from the Biometrics Research Department at New York State Psychiatric Institute, Unit 60, 1051 Riverside Drive, New York, NY 10032; 212-543-5524. Refer to the SCID-CV User's Guide for a discussion of the differences between the Research Version and the Clinician Version of the SCID. For up-to-date information about the SCID, including information about training and computerized versions, please visit our web site: www.scid4.org.

OVERVIEW

I'm going to be asking you about problems or difficulties you may have had, and I'll be making some notes as we go along. Do you have any questions before we begin?

(ADMINISTER OVERVIEW QUESTIONS ON SCORESHEET.)

A. MOOD EPISODES

MAJOR DEPRESSIVE EPISODE

Now I am going to ask you some more questions about your mood.

A1 In the past month. . .

. . .has there been a period of time when you were feeling depressed or down most of the day, nearly every day? (What was that like?)

IF YES: How long did it last? (As long as 2 weeks?)

A2 . . .what about losing interest or pleasure in things you usually enjoyed?

IF YES: Was it nearly every day? How long did it last? (As long as 2 weeks?)

CRITERIA FOR MAJOR DEPRESSIVE EPISODE

NOTE: Criterion B (i.e., does not meet criteria for a Mixed Episode) has been omitted from the SCID.

A. Five (or more) of the following symptoms have been present during the same 2-week period and represent a change from previous functioning; at least one of the symptoms is either (1) depressed mood or (2) loss of interest or pleasure

(1) depressed mood most of the day, nearly every day, as indicated by either subjective report (e.g., feels sad or empty) or observation made by others (e.g., appears tearful). **Note:** In children and adolescents, can be irritable mood. **A1**

(2) markedly diminished interest or pleasure in all, or almost all, activities most of the day, nearly every day (as indicated by either subjective account or observation made by others) **A2**

If **<u>neither</u> A1 <u>nor</u> A2** is "+" during the current month, check for past Major Depressive Episode by asking questions A1 and A2 again looking for lifetime episodes, beginning with "Has there EVER. . ."

IF AT LEAST ONE PAST DEPRESSED PERIOD: Have you had more than one time like that? Which one was the worst?

If **<u>neither</u> A1 <u>nor</u> A2** has ever been "+," go to **A16**, page 8 *(Manic Episode).*

FOR THE FOLLOWING QUESTIONS, FOCUS ON THE WORST 2-WEEK PERIOD:

During [2-WEEK PERIOD] . . .

A3 . . . how was your appetite? (What about compared with your usual appetite? Did you have to force yourself to eat? Eat [less/more] than usual? Was that nearly every day? Did you lose or gain any weight? How much? Were you trying to lose weight?)

(3) significant weight loss when not dieting or weight gain (e.g., a change of more than 5% of body weight in a month), or decrease or increase in appetite nearly every day. **Note:** In children, consider failure to make expected weight gains. **A3**

A4 . . . how were you sleeping? (Trouble falling asleep, waking frequently, trouble staying asleep, waking too early, OR sleeping too much? How many hours a night compared with usual? Was that nearly every night?)

(4) insomnia or hypersomnia nearly every day **A4**

A5 . . . were you so fidgety or restless that you were unable to sit still? (Was it so bad that other people noticed it? What did they notice? Was that nearly every day?)

IF NO: What about the opposite—talking or moving more slowly than is normal for you? (Was it so bad that other people noticed it? What did they notice? Was that nearly every day?)

(5) psychomotor agitation or retardation nearly every day (observable by others, not merely subjective feelings of restlessness or being slowed down) **A5**

NOTE: ALSO CONSIDER BEHAVIOR DURING THE INTERVIEW

A6 . . . what was your energy like? (Tired all the time? Nearly every day?)

(6) fatigue or loss of energy nearly every day **A6**

A7 . . . how did you feel about yourself? (Worthless? Nearly every day?)

. . . what about feeling guilty about things you had done or not done? (Nearly every day?)

(7) feelings of worthlessness or excessive or inappropriate guilt (which may be delusional) nearly every day (not merely self-reproach or guilt about being sick) **A7**

NOTE: CODE "–" IF ONLY LOW SELF-ESTEEM

A8 . . . did you have trouble thinking or concentrating? (What kinds of things did it interfere with? Nearly every day?)

IF NO: Was it hard to make decisions about everyday things?

(8) diminished ability to think or concentrate, or indecisiveness, nearly every day (either by objective account or as observed by others) **A8**

A9 . . . were things so bad that you were thinking a lot about death or that you would be better off dead? What about thinking of hurting yourself?

IF YES: Did you do anything to hurt yourself?

(9) recurrent thoughts of death (not just fear of dying), recurrent suicidal ideation without a specific plan, or a suicide attempt or a specific plan for committing suicide **A9**

A10 **AT LEAST FIVE OF A(1)–A(9) ARE "+" AND AT LEAST ONE OF THESE IS ITEM A(1) OR A(2).** **A10**

If **A10** above is "—" (i.e., fewer than five are "+"), ask the following if unknown:

Have there been any other times when you've been depressed and had even more of the symptoms that we've just talked about?

If "yes," go back to **A1,** page 3, and ask about that episode.
If "no," go to **A16,** page 8 *(Manic Episode)*.

A11 IF UNCLEAR: Has [the depression/OWN WORDS] made it hard for you to do your work, take care of things at home, or get along with other people?

C. The symptoms cause clinically significant distress or impairment in social, occupational, or other important areas of functioning. **A11**

If **A11** above is "–" (i.e., symptoms not clinically significant), ask the following if unknown:

Have there been any <u>other</u> times when you've been depressed and it had more of an effect on your life?

If "yes," go back to **A1**, page 3, and ask about that episode.
If "no," go to **A16**, page 8 (*Manic Episode).*

A12 Just before this began, were you physically ill?

Just before this began, were you taking any medications?

IF YES: Any change in the amount you were taking?

Just before this began, were you drinking or using any street drugs?

If there is any indication that the depression may be secondary (i.e., a direct physiological consequence of a general medical condition or substance), go to page 20 and return here to make a rating of "–" or "+."

D. The symptoms are not due to the direct physiological effects of a substance (e.g., a drug of abuse, medication) or a general medical condition. **A12**

<u>Etiological general medical conditions include</u> degenerative neurological illnesses (e.g., Parkinson's disease), cerebrovascular disease (e.g., stroke), metabolic conditions (e.g., vitamin B_{12} deficiency), endocrine conditions (e.g., hyper- and hypothyroidism, hyper- and hypoadrenocorticism), viral or other infections (e.g., hepatitis, mononucleosis, HIV), and certain cancers (e.g., carcinoma of the pancreas).

<u>Etiological substances include</u> alcohol, amphetamines, cocaine, hallucinogens, inhalants, opioids, phencyclidine, sedatives, hypnotics, anxiolytics. Medications include antihypertensives, oral contraceptives, corticosteroids, anabolic steroids, anticancer agents, analgesics, anticholinergics, cardiac medications.

If **A12** above is "–" (i.e., mood <u>is</u> due to substance or general medical condition), ask the following:

Have there been any <u>other</u> times when you've been depressed and it was not because of [GENERAL MEDICAL CONDITION/SUBSTANCE USE]?

If "yes," go back to **A1**, page 3, and ask about that episode.
If "no," go to **A16**, page 8 (*Manic Episode*).

A13 IF UNKNOWN: Did this begin soon after someone close to you died?

E. The symptoms are not better accounted for by Bereavement, i.e., after the loss [death] of a loved one, the symptoms persist for longer than 2 months or are characterized by marked functional impairment, morbid preoccupation with worthlessness, suicidal ideation, psychotic symptoms, or psychomotor retardation. **A13**

If **A13** above is "–" (i.e., the depressed mood is better accounted for by Bereavement), ask the following:

Have there been any other times when you've been depressed and it was not because of the loss of a loved one?

If "yes," go back to **A1**, page 3, and ask about that episode.
If "no," go to **A16**, page 8 (*Manic Episode*).

A14 IF UNKNOWN: Have you had (SYMPTOMS RATED "+" ABOVE) in the past month?

CRITERIA A, C, D, AND E ARE "+" **A14**

(MAKE A DIAGNOSIS OF MAJOR DEPRESSIVE EPISODE)

A15 How many separate times have you been [depressed/OWN WORDS] nearly every day for at least 2 weeks and had several of the symptoms that you just described, such as [SYMPTOMS OF WORST EPISODE]?

Total number of Major Depressive Episodes, including current (CODE 99 if too numerous or indistinct to count) **A15**

MANIC EPISODE

CRITERIA FOR MANIC EPISODE

NOTE: Criterion C (i.e., does not meet criteria for a Mixed Episode) has been omitted from the SCID.

A16 Have you ever had a period of time when you were feeling so good, high, excited, or hyper that other people thought you were not your normal self or you got into trouble? (Did anyone say you were manic? Was that more than just feeling good?)

What was that like?

IF NO: What about a period of time when you were so irritable that you found yourself shouting at people or starting fights or arguments? (Did you find yourself yelling at people you didn't really know?)

A. A distinct period of abnormally and persistently elevated, expansive, or irritable mood. . . **A16**

If **A16** is "–" (i.e., never any periods of elevated or irritable mood), go to **A45**, page 17 (*Dysthymic Disorder*).

A17 How long did that last? (As long as 1 week? Did you have to go into the hospital?)

. . . lasting at least 1 week (or any duration if hospitalization is necessary) **A17**

If **A17** is "–" (i.e., duration is less than 1 week), go to **A30**, page 13 (*Hypomanic Episode*).

Have you had more than one time such as that? Which time were you the most [high/irritable/OWN WORDS?]

FOR ITEMS **A18–A27** ON PAGES 9–11, FOCUS ON THE MOST EXTREME EPISODE

IF UNKNOWN: During this time, when were you the most [OWN WORDS for euphoria or irritability]?

	Interview question	Criterion	
	During [PERIOD OF WORST MANIC SYMPTOMS]...	B. During the period of mood disturbance, three (or more) of the following symptoms have persisted (four if the mood is only irritable) and have been present to a significant degree:	
A18	...how did you feel about yourself? (More self-confident than usual? Any special powers or abilities?)	(1) inflated self-esteem or grandiosity	**A18**
A19	...did you need less sleep than usual? IF YES: Did you still feel rested?	(2) decreased need for sleep (e.g., feels rested after only 3 hours of sleep)	**A19**
A20	...were you much more talkative than usual? (Did people have trouble stopping you or understanding you? Did people have trouble getting a word in edgewise?)	(3) more talkative than usual or pressure to keep talking	**A20**
A21	...were your thoughts racing through your head?	(4) flight of ideas or subjective experience that thoughts are racing	**A21**
A22	...were you so easily distracted by things around you that you had trouble concentrating or staying on one track?	(5) distractibility (i.e., attention too easily drawn to unimportant or irrelevant external stimuli)	**A22**
A23	...how did you spend your time? (Work, friends, hobbies? Were you so active that your friends or family were concerned about you?) IF NO INCREASED ACTIVITY: Were you physically restless? (How bad was it?)	(6) increase in goal-directed activity (socially, at work or school, or sexually) or psychomotor agitation	**A23**

A24 . . .did you do anything that could have caused trouble for you or your family? (Buying things you didn't need? Anything sexual that was unusual for you? Reckless driving?)

(7) excessive involvement in pleasurable activities that have a high potential for painful consequences (e.g., engaging in unrestrained buying sprees, sexual indiscretions, or foolish business investments) **A24**

A25

AT LEAST THREE OF B(1)–B(7) ARE "+" (OR FOUR IF MOOD IS IRRITABLE AND NOT ELEVATED) **A25**

If **A25** above is "–" (i.e., fewer than three are "+") ask the following:

Have there been any other times when you were [high/irritable/OWN WORDS] and had even more of the symptoms that we've just talked about?

If "yes," go back to **A16**, page 8, and ask about that episode.
If "no," go to **A45**, page 17 *(Dysthymic Disorder).*

A26 IF NOT KNOWN: At that time, did you have serious problems at home or at work (school) because you were [SYMPTOMS] or did you have to go into a hospital?

D. The mood disturbance is sufficiently severe to cause marked impairment in occupational functioning or in usual social activities or relationships with others, or to necessitate hospitalization to prevent harm to self or others, or there are psychotic features. **A26**

If **A26** above is "–" (i.e., not sufficiently severe) ask the following:

Have there been any other times when you were [high/irritable/OWN WORDS] and you got into trouble with people or were hospitalized?

If "yes," go back to **A16**, page 8, and ask about that episode.
If "no," go to **A39**, page 14 *(Criterion C for Hypomanic Episode).*

A27 Just before this began, were you physically ill?

Just before this began, were you taking any medications?

IF YES: Any change in the amount you were taking?

Just before this began, were you drinking or using any street drugs?

If there is any indication that the mania may be secondary (i.e., a direct physiological consequence of a general medical condition or substance), go to page 20 and return here to make a rating of "–" or "+."

E. The symptoms are not due to the direct physiological effects of a substance (e.g., a drug of abuse, a medication) or a general medical condition. **A27**

Note: Manic-like episodes that are clearly caused by somatic antidepressant treatment (e.g., medication, electroconvulsive therapy, light therapy) should not count toward a diagnosis of Bipolar I Disorder but are considered Substance-Induced Mood Disorders.

<u>Etiological general medical conditions include</u> degenerative neurological illnesses (e.g., Huntington's disease, multiple sclerosis), cerebrovascular disease (e.g., stroke), metabolic conditions (e.g., vitamin B_{12} deficiency, Wilson's disease), endocrine conditions (e.g., hyperthyroidism), viral or other infections, and certain cancers (e.g., cerebral neoplasms).

<u>Etiological substances include</u> alcohol, amphetamines, cocaine, hallucinogens, inhalants, opioids, phencyclidine, sedatives, hypnotics, and anxiolytics. Medications include psychotropic medications (e.g., antidepressants), corticosteroids, anabolic steroids, isoniazid, antiparkinson medication (e.g., levodopa), and sympathomimetics/ decongestants.

If **A27** above is "–" (i.e., the mania is due to a substance or general medical condition), ask the following:

Have there been any other times when you were [high/irritable/OWN WORDS] and you were not [physically ill/taking medication/using SUBSTANCE]?

If "yes," go back to **A16**, page 8, and ask about that episode.
If "no," go to **A45**, page 17 *(Dysthymic Disorder)*.

A28	IF UNKNOWN: Have you had [SYMPTOMS RATED "+" ABOVE] in the past month?	**CRITERIA A, C, D, AND E ARE "+"** (MAKE A DIAGNOSIS OF MANIC EPISODE)	**A28**
A29	How many separate times were you [HIGH/OWN WORDS] and had [ACKNOWLEDGED MANIC SYMPTOMS] for at least a week (or were hospitalized)?	Total number of Manic Episodes, including current (CODE 99 if too indistinct or numerous to count)	**A29**

YOU ARE FINISHED EVALUATING MOOD EPISODES. GO TO MODULE B (PSYCHOTIC AND ASSOCIATED SYMPTOMS), **B1** (PAGE 25).

HYPOMANIC EPISODE

A30 IF UNKNOWN: When you were [high/irritable/OWN WORDS], did it last for at least 4 days?

Have you had more than one time like that? (Which time were you the most [high/irritable/OWN WORDS]?)

FOR ITEMS **A31–A37** ON PAGES 13 AND 14, FOCUS ON THE MOST EXTREME EPISODE

CRITERIA FOR HYPOMANIC EPISODE

A. A distinct period of persistently elevated, expansive, or irritable mood, lasting throughout at least 4 days, that is clearly different from the usual nondepressed mood. **A30**

If **A30** is "–" (i.e., never any periods of elevated or irritable mood lasting at least 4 days), go to **A45**, page 17 (*Dysthymic Disorder*).

During [PERIOD OF MOST EXTREME HYPOMANIC SYMPTOMS]...

B. During the period of mood disturbance, three (or more) of the following symptoms have persisted (four if the mood is only irritable) and have been present to a significant degree:

A31 ...how did you feel about yourself?

(More self-confident than usual? Any special powers or abilities?)

(1) inflated self-esteem or grandiosity **A31**

A32 ...did you need less sleep than usual?

IF YES: Did you still feel rested?

(2) decreased need for sleep (e.g., feels rested after only 3 hours of sleep) **A32**

A33 ...were you much more talkative than usual? (Did people have trouble stopping you or understanding you? Did people have trouble getting a word in edgewise?)

(3) more talkative than usual or pressure to keep talking **A33**

A34 ...were your thoughts racing through your head?

(4) flight of ideas or subjective experience that thoughts are racing **A34**

A35 ...were you so easily distracted by things around you that you had trouble concentrating or staying on one track?

(5) distractibility (i.e., attention too easily drawn to unimportant or irrelevant external stimuli) **A35**

A36 . . .how did you spend your time? (Work, friends, hobbies? Were you so active that your friends or family were concerned about you?)

IF NO INCREASED ACTIVITY: Were you physically restless? (How bad was it?)

(6) increase in goal-directed activity (either socially, at work or school, or sexually) or psychomotor agitation **A36**

A37 . . .did you do anything that could have caused trouble for you or your family? (Buying things you didn't need? Anything sexual that was unusual for you? Reckless driving?)

(7) excessive involvement in pleasurable activities that have a high potential for painful consequences (e.g., engaging in unrestrained buying sprees, sexual indiscretions, or foolish business investments) **A37**

A38

AT LEAST THREE OF B(1)–B(7) ARE "+" (OR FOUR IF MOOD IS IRRITABLE AND NOT ELEVATED) **A38**

If **A38** is "–" (i.e., fewer than three are "+"), ask the following:

Have there been any <u>other</u> times when you were [high/irritable/OWN WORDS] and had even more of the symptoms that we've just talked about?

If "yes," go back to **A30**, page 13, and ask about that episode.
If "no," go to **A45**, page 17 (*Dysthymic Disorder*).

A39 IF UNKNOWN: Is this very different from the way you usually are? (How were you different? At work? With friends?)

C. The episode is associated with an unequivocal change in functioning that is uncharacteristic of the person when not symptomatic. **A39**

If **A39** is "–" (i.e., characteristically "hypomanic"), ask the following:

Have there been any <u>other</u> times when you were [high/irritable/OWN WORDS] and you were really different from the way you usually are?

If "yes," go back to **A30**, page 13, and ask about that episode.
If "no," go to **A45**, page 17 (*Dysthymic Disorder*).

A40 IF UNKNOWN: Did other people notice the change in you? (What did they say?)

D. The disturbance in mood and the change in functioning are observable by others. **A40**

If **A40** is "–" (i.e., not observable by others), ask the following:

Have there been any <u>other</u> times when you were [high/irritable/OWN WORDS] and other people <u>did</u> notice the change in the way you were acting?

If "yes," go back to **A30,** page 13, and ask about that episode.
If "no," go to **A45,** page 17 *(Dysthymic Disorder).*

A41 IF UNKNOWN: At that time, did you have serious problems at home or at work (school) because you were [SYMPTOMS] or did you have to go into a hospital?

E. The episode is not severe enough to cause marked impairment in social or occupational functioning, or to necessitate hospitalization, and there are no psychotic features. **A41**

If **A41** is "–" (i.e., severe enough to cause marked impairment, etc.) AND either hospitalization was required or duration was 1 week or longer, go back to **A17,** page 8, and recode "+" for that item, then continue with the rest of the ratings for Manic Episode. Otherwise, if there was marked impairment in functioning but duration was less than 1 week, skip to **A45,** page 17, and eventually code "2" for item **D12,** page 49.

A42 Just before this began, were you physically ill?

Just before this began, were you taking any medications?

IF YES: Any change in the amount you were taking?

Just before this began, were you drinking or using any street drugs?

If there is any indication that the hypomania may be secondary (i.e., a direct physiological consequence of a general medical condition or substance), go to page 20 and return here to make a rating of "–" or "+."

F. The symptoms are not due to the direct physiological effects of a substance (i.e., a drug of abuse, a medication) or a general medical condition. **A42**

Note: Hypomanic-like episodes that are clearly caused by somatic antidepressant treatment (e.g., medication, electroconvulsive therapy, light therapy) should not count toward a diagnosis of Bipolar II Disorder but are considered Substance-Induced Mood Episodes.

*Refer to list of possibly etiological general medical conditions and substances included with item **A27** (page 11).*

If **A42** above is "–" (i.e., the hypomania is due to a substance or general medical condition), ask the following:

Have there been any other times when you were [high/irritable/OWN WORDS] and you were not [physically ill/taking medication/using SUBSTANCE]?

If "yes," go back to **A30**, page 13, and ask about that episode.
If "no," go to **A45**, page 17 *(Dysthymic Disorder).*

A43	IF UNKNOWN: Have you had [SYMPTOMS RATED "+" ABOVE] in the past month?	**CRITERIA A, B, C, D, E, AND F ARE "+"** (MAKE A DIAGNOSIS OF HYPOMANIC EPISODE)	**A43**
A44	How many separate times were you [high/irritable/OWN WORDS] and had [ACKNOWLEDGED HYPOMANIC SYMPTOMS] for a period of time?	Total number of Hypomanic Episodes (CODE 99 if too indistinct or numerous to count)	**A44**

YOU ARE FINISHED EVALUATING MOOD EPISODES. GO TO MODULE B (PSYCHOTIC AND ASSOCIATED SYMPTOMS), **B1** (PAGE 25).

DYSTHYMIC DISORDER		**CRITERIA FOR DYSTHYMIC DISORDER**	
	NOTE: For presentations in which there is a history of multiple recurrent Major Depressive Episodes, the clinician may wish to skip the evaluation of Dysthymic Disorder (i.e., go to **B1**, page 25).		
A45	For the past couple of years, have you been bothered by depressed mood, most of the day, more days than not? (more than half the time?) IF YES: What was that like?	A. Depressed mood for most of the day, for more days than not, as indicated either by subjective account or observation by others, for at least 2 years. **Note:** In children and adolescents, mood can be irritable and duration must be at least 1 year.	**A45**

If **A45** is "–" (i.e., no chronic depressed mood...), go to **B1**, page 25 *(Psychotic and Associated Symptoms)*.

	During these periods of [OWN WORDS FOR CHRONIC DEPRESSION], do you find that most of the time you...	B. Presence, while depressed, of two (or more) of the following:	
A46	...lose your appetite? (What about overeating?)	(1) poor appetite or overeating	**A46**
A47	...have trouble sleeping or sleep too much?	(2) insomnia or hypersomnia	**A47**
A48	...have little energy to do things or feel tired a lot?	(3) low energy or fatigue	**A48**
A49	...feel down on yourself? (Feel worthless, or a failure?)	(4) low self-esteem	**A49**
A50	...have trouble concentrating or making decisions?	(5) poor concentration or difficulty making decisions	**A50**
A51	...feel hopeless?	(6) feelings of hopelessness	**A51**
A52		**AT LEAST TWO "B" SYMPTOMS ARE "+"**	**A52**

If **A52** is "–" (i.e., fewer than two symptoms are "+"), go to **B1**, page 25 *(Psychotic and Associated Symptoms)*.

A53 What is the longest time, during this period of long-lasting depression, that you felt OK? (NO DYSTHYMIC SYMPTOMS)

C. During the 2-year period (1 year for children or adolescents) of the disturbance, the person has never been without the symptoms in criteria A and B for more than 2 months at a time. **A53**

If **A53** is "–" (i.e., more than 2 months without symptoms), go to **B1**, page 25 *(Psychotic and Associated Symptoms)*.

A54 How long have you been feeling this way? (When did this begin?)

Age at onset of current Dysthymic Disorder (CODE 99 IF UNKNOWN) **A54**

A55 IF UNKNOWN: Did it begin gradually or did it start with a bad period of depression?

D. No Major Depressive Episode during the first 2 years of the disturbance (1 year for children and adolescents); i.e., not better accounted for by chronic Major Depressive Disorder, or Major Depressive Disorder, In Partial Remission **A55**

Note: There may have been a previous Major Depressive Episode provided there was a full remission (no significant signs or symptoms for 2 months) before development of the Dysthymic Disorder. In addition, after the initial 2 years (1 year in children or adolescents) of Dysthymic Disorder, there may be superimposed episodes of Major Depressive Disorder, in which case both diagnoses may be given when the criteria are met for a Major Depressive Episode.

If **A55** is "–" (i.e., Major Depressive Episode during first 2 years), go to **B1**, page 25 *(Psychotic and Associated Symptoms)*.

A56

E. There has never been a Manic Episode, a Mixed Episode, or a Hypomanic Episode, and criteria have never been met for Cyclothymic Disorder. **A56**

If **A56** is "–" (i.e., past Manic, Mixed, or Hypomanic Episode or criteria met for Cyclothymic Disorder), go to **B1**, page 25 *(Psychotic and Associated Symptoms)*.

A57 THIS MAY NEED TO BE DEFERRED UNTIL AFTER PSYCHOTIC DISORDERS HAVE BEEN RULED OUT.

F. Does not occur exclusively during the course of a chronic Psychotic Disorder, such as Schizophrenia or Delusional Disorder. **A57**

> If **A57** is "–" (i.e., occurs during Psychotic Disorder), go to **B1**, page 25 *(Psychotic and Associated Symptoms)*.

A58 Just before this began, were you physically ill?

Just before this began, were you taking any medications?

IF YES: Any change in the amount you were taking?

Just before this began, were you drinking or using any street drugs?

> If there is any indication that the dysthymia may be secondary (i.e., a direct physiological consequence of a general medical condition or substance), go to page 20 and return here to make a rating of "–" or "+."

G. The symptoms are not due to the direct physiological effects of a substance (e.g., a drug of abuse, a medication) or a general medical condition. **A58**

Etiological general medical conditions include degenerative neurological illnesses (e.g., Parkinson's disease), cerebrovascular disease (e.g., stroke), metabolic conditions (e.g., vitamin B_{12} deficiency), endocrine conditions (e.g., hyper- and hypothyroidism, hyper- and hypoadrenocorticism), viral or other infections (e.g., hepatitis, mononucleosis, HIV), and certain cancers (e.g., carcinoma of the pancreas).

Etiological substances include alcohol, amphetamines, cocaine, hallucinogens, inhalants, opioids, phencyclidine, sedatives, hypnotics, anxiolytics. Medications include antihypertensives, oral contraceptives, corticosteroids, anabolic steroids, anticancer agents, analgesics, anticholinergics, and cardiac medications.

> If **A58** is "–" (i.e., due to a chronic general medical condition or chronic substance use), go to **B1**, page 25 *(Psychotic and Associated Symptoms)*.

A59 IF UNCLEAR: How much do [SYMPTOMS IN A AND B] interfere with your life?

H. The symptoms cause clinically significant distress or impairment in social, occupational, or other important areas of functioning. **A59**

> If **A59** is "–" (i.e., not clinically significant), go to **B1**, page 25 *(Psychotic and Associated Symptoms)*.

A60

CRITERIA A, B, C, D, E, F, G, AND H ARE "+" **A60**

(MAKE A DIAGNOSIS OF 300.4 DYSTHYMIC DISORDER)

> Go to **B1**, page 25 *(Psychotic and Associated Symptoms)*.

CONSIDER ETIOLOGICAL ROLE OF A GENERAL MEDICAL CONDITION OR SUBSTANCE USE

If mood symptoms are not temporally associated with a general medical condition, go to **A65**, page 22 (*Substance-Induced Mood Disorder*).

MOOD DISORDER DUE TO A GENERAL MEDICAL CONDITION

CRITERIA FOR MOOD DISORDER DUE TO A GENERAL MEDICAL CONDITION

NOTE: Criterion D (i.e., not during delirium) has been omitted from the SCID.

A61 CODE BASED ON INFORMATION ALREADY OBTAINED

A. A prominent and persistent disturbance in mood predominant in the clinical picture and by either (or both) of the following: **A61**

(1) depressed mood or markedly diminished interest or pleasure in all, or almost all, activities

(2) elevated, expansive, or irritable mood

A62 Do you think your [MOOD SYMPTOMS] were in any way related to your [COMORBID GENERAL MEDICAL CONDITION]?

IF YES: Tell me how.

(Did the [MOOD SYMPTOMS] start or get much worse only after [COMORBID GENERAL MEDICAL CONDITION] began?)

IF YES AND GENERAL MEDICAL CONDITION HAS RESOLVED: Did the [MOOD SYMPTOMS] get better once the [COMORBID GENERAL MEDICAL CONDITION] got better?

B/C. There is evidence from the history, physical examination, or laboratory findings that the disturbance is the direct physiological consequence of a general medical condition, and the disturbance is not better accounted for by another mental disorder (e.g., Adjustment Disorder With Depressed Mood in response to the stress of having a general medical condition). **A62**

If **A62** is "–" (general medical condition not etiological), go to **A65**, page 22 (*Substance-Induced Mood Disorder*).

A63 IF UNCLEAR: How much did [MOOD SYMPTOMS] interfere with your life?

E. The symptoms cause clinically significant distress or impairment in social, occupational, or other important areas of functioning. **A63**

A64 IF UNKNOWN: Have you had [SYMPTOMS RATED "+" ABOVE] in the past month?

CRITERIA A, B/C, AND E ARE "+" **A64**

(MAKE A DIAGNOSIS OF 293.83 MOOD DISORDER DUE TO A GENERAL MEDICAL CONDITION)

If mood symptoms are <u>not</u> temporally associated with substance use, return to episode being evaluated:

A12 for Major Depressive Episode (page 6)
A27 for Manic Episode (page 11)
A42 for Hypomanic Episode (page 15)
A58 for Dysthymic Disorder (page 19)
D11 for Other Bipolar Disorders (page 49)
D18 for Depressive Disorder NOS (page 52)

SUBSTANCE-INDUCED MOOD DISORDER

CRITERIA FOR SUBSTANCE-INDUCED MOOD DISORDER

NOTE: Criterion D (i.e., not due to delirium) has been omitted from the SCID.

A65 CODE BASED ON INFORMATION ALREADY OBTAINED

A. A prominent and persistent disturbance in mood predominant in the clinical picture and characterized by either (or both) of the following: **A65**

(1) depressed or markedly diminished interest or pleasure in all, or almost all, activities

(2) elevated, expansive, or irritable mood

A66 IF UNKNOWN: When did the [MOOD SYMPTOMS] begin? Were you already using [SUBSTANCE] or had you just stopped or cut down your use?

B. There is evidence from the history, physical examination, or laboratory findings of either (1) or (2) **A66**

(1) the symptoms in criterion A developed during, or within a month of, Substance Intoxication or Withdrawal

(2) medication use is etiologically related to the disturbance

If **A66** is "–" (i.e., not etiologically related to a substance), then return to episode being evaluated:

A12 for Major Depressive Episode (page 6)
A27 for Manic Episode (page 11)
A42 for Hypomanic Episode (page 15)
A58 for Dysthymic Disorder (page 19)
D11 for Other Bipolar Disorders (page 49)
D18 for Depressive Disorder NOS (page 52)

A67 Do you think your [MOOD SYMPTOMS] are in any way related to your [SUBSTANCE USE]?

IF YES: Tell me how.

ASK ANY OF THE FOLLOWING QUESTIONS AS NEEDED TO RULE OUT A NONSUBSTANCE ETIOLOGY

C. The disturbance is not better accounted for by a Mood Disorder that is not substance induced. Evidence that the symptoms are better accounted for by a Mood Disorder that is not substance induced might include: **A67**

A67 (cont'd)

IF UNKNOWN: Which came first, the [SUBSTANCE USE] or the [MOOD SYMPTOMS]?

(1) the mood symptoms precede the onset of the substance use (or medication use)

IF UNKNOWN: Have you had a period of time when you stopped using [SUBSTANCE]?

IF YES: After you stopped using [SUBSTANCE] did the [MOOD SYMPTOMS] get better?

(2) the mood symptoms persist for a substantial period of time (e.g., about a month) after the cessation of acute withdrawal or severe intoxication

IF UNKNOWN: How much of [SUBSTANCE] were you using when you began to have [MOOD SYMPTOMS]?

(3) the mood symptoms are substantially in excess of what would be expected given the type or amount of the substance used or the duration of use

IF UNKNOWN: Have you had any other episodes of [MOOD SYMPTOMS]?

IF YES: How many? Were you using [SUBSTANCE] at those times?

(4) there is other evidence that suggests the existence of an independent non-substance-induced Mood Disorder (e.g., a history of recurrent non-substance-related Major Depressive Episodes)

If **A67** is "–" (i.e., the disturbance is better accounted for by a non-substance-induced Mood Disorder), then return to episode being evaluated:

A12 for Major Depressive Episode (page 6)
A27 for Manic Episode (page 11)
A42 for Hypomanic Episode (page 15)
A58 for Dysthymic Disorder (page 19)
D11 for Other Bipolar Disorders (page 49)
D18 for Depressive Disorder NOS (page 52)

A68

IF UNKNOWN: How much did [MOOD SYMPTOMS] interfere with your life?

E. The symptoms cause clinically significant distress or impairment in social, occupational, or other important areas of functioning.

A69

IF UNKNOWN: Have you had [SYMPTOMS RATED "+" ABOVE] in the past month?

CRITERIA A, B, C, AND E ARE "+"

(MAKE A DIAGNOSIS OF SUBSTANCE-INDUCED MOOD DISORDER)

Return to episode being evaluated:

A12 for Major Depressive Episode (page 6)
A27 for Manic Episode (page 11)
A42 for Hypomanic Episode (page 15)
A58 for Dysthymic Disorder (page 19)
D11 for Other Bipolar Disorders (page 49)
D18 for Depressive Disorder NOS (page 52)

B. PSYCHOTIC AND ASSOCIATED SYMPTOMS

FOR EACH PSYCHOTIC SYMPTOM, DESCRIBE ON THE SCORESHEET THE ACTUAL CONTENT AND INDICATE THE PERIOD OF TIME DURING WHICH THE SYMPTOM WAS PRESENT.

Now I am going to ask you about unusual experiences that people sometimes have.

DELUSIONS

False personal beliefs based on incorrect inference about external reality and firmly sustained in spite of what almost everyone else believes and in spite of what constitutes incontrovertible and obvious proof or evidence to the contrary. The belief is not one ordinarily accepted by other members of the person's culture or subculture. Do not consider as delusions unreasonable and sustained beliefs that are maintained with less than delusional intensity ("overvalued ideas").

B1 Has it ever seemed like people were talking about you or taking special notice of you?

IF YES: Were you convinced they were talking about you, or did you think it might have been your imagination?

Delusion of reference; i.e., events, objects, or other people in the individual's environment have a particular or unusual significance that is clearly unwarranted. **B1**

B2 What about anyone going out of his or her way to give you a hard time, or trying to hurt you?

Persecutory delusion; i.e., the individual (or his or her group) is being attacked, cheated, persecuted, or conspired against. **B2**

B3	Did you ever feel that you were especially important in some way, or that you had special powers to do things that other people couldn't do?	Grandiose delusion; i.e., content involves exaggerated power, knowledge, or importance, or a special relationship to a deity or famous person.	**B3**
B4	Did you ever feel that something was very wrong with you physically even though your doctor said nothing was wrong . . . like you had cancer or some other terrible disease? Have you ever been convinced that something was very wrong with the way a part or parts of your body looked? (Did you ever feel that something strange was happening to parts of your body?)	Somatic delusion; i.e., content involves change or disturbance in body appearance or functioning.	**B4**
B5	(Did you ever have any unusual religious experiences?) (Did you ever feel that you had committed a crime or done something terrible for which you should be punished?) (Did you ever feel that someone or something outside yourself was controlling your thoughts or actions against your will?) (Did you ever believe that someone could read your mind?) (Did you ever feel that certain thoughts that were not your own were put into your head? What about taken out of your head?)	Other delusions; i.e., religious, jealous, erotomanic, delusions of guilt, delusions of being controlled, thought broadcasting, thought insertion, thought withdrawal.	**B5**

HALLUCINATIONS

A sensory perception that has the compelling sense of reality of a true perception but occurs without external stimulation of the relevant sensory organ.

B6	Did you hear things that other people couldn't hear, such as noises, or the voices of people whispering or talking? IF YES: What did you hear? How often did you hear it?	Auditory hallucinations when fully awake, heard either inside or outside the head.	**B6**
B7	Did you ever have visions or see things that other people couldn't see? (Were you awake at the time?)	Visual hallucinations.	**B7**
B8	What about strange sensations in your body or on your skin?	Tactile hallucinations, e.g., electricity.	**B8**
B9	What about smelling or tasting things that other people couldn't smell or taste? THE REMAINDER OF THE ITEMS IN THIS SECTION ARE OBSERVATIONAL OR BY HISTORY Let me stop for a minute while I make a few notes.	Other hallucinations, e.g., gustatory, olfactory.	**B9**
B10		Catatonic behaviors; e.g., catalepsy, stupor, catatonic agitation, negativism, mutism, posturing, stereotyped movements, echolalia, echopraxia.	**B10**

B11		Grossly disorganized behavior; e.g., markedly disheveled appearance, grossly inappropriate sexual behavior, unpredictable or untriggered agitation.	B11
B12		Grossly inappropriate affect; e.g., smiling while discussing being persecuted.	B12
B13		Disorganized speech; e.g., frequent derailment (loosening of associations) or incoherence.	B13
B14		Negative symptoms; i.e., affective flattening, alogia, avolition.	B14
B15	IF DELUSIONS OR HALLUCINATIONS HAVE EVER BEEN PRESENT, FILL OUT CHRONOLOGY SECTION.		B15

C. DIFFERENTIAL DIAGNOSIS OF PSYCHOTIC DISORDERS

If no psychotic items from Module B have ever been present, go to **Module D,** page 45 *(Mood Disorders).*

C1 Psychotic symptoms occur at times other than during Major Depressive, Manic, and Mixed Episodes. **C1**

The following question may be asked for clarification: IF A MAJOR DEPRESSIVE, MANIC, OR MIXED EPISODE HAS EVER BEEN PRESENT: Has there ever been a time when you had [PSYCHOTIC SYMPTOMS] and you were not [DEPRESSED/MANIC]?

yes ↓

no → Psychotic Mood— Go to **Module D,** page 45

CRITERIA FOR SCHIZOPHRENIA

NOTE: Criteria for Schizophrenia are presented in a different order than in DSM-IV.

C2 A. Two (or more) of the following, each present for a significant portion of time during a 1-month period (or less if successfully treated): **C2**

(1) delusions

(2) hallucinations

(3) disorganized speech (e.g., frequent derailment or incoherence)

(4) grossly disorganized or catatonic behavior

(5) negative symptoms i.e., affective flattening, alogia, or avolition

[**Note:** Only one criterion A symptom is required if delusions are bizarre or hallucinations consist of a voice keeping up a running commentary on the person's behavior or thoughts, or two or more voices conversing with each other.]

yes ↓

no → Go to **C21,** page 36

C3

D. Schizoaffective Disorder and Mood Disorder With Psychotic Features have been ruled out because either:

(1) no Major Depressive, Manic, or Mixed Episodes have occurred concurrently with the active-phase symptoms (i.e., the "A" symptoms listed in C2).

The following question may be asked for clarification: Has there ever been a time when you had [PSYCHOTIC SYMPTOMS] at the same time that you were [depressed/high/irritable/OWN WORDS]?

(2) if mood episodes have occurred concurrently during active-phase symptoms, their total duration has been brief relative to the duration of the active and residual periods.

Question for clarification: How much of the time that you have had [SYMPTOMS FROM ACTIVE AND RESIDUAL PHASES] would you say you have also been [depressed/high/irritable/OWN WORDS]?

NOTE: Answer "yes" if there have never been any Major Depressive, Manic, or Mixed Episodes, if all such episodes occurred during the prodromal or residual phase, or if mood symptoms are brief relative to the total disturbance. Answer "no" if any mood episodes overlap with psychotic symptoms AND the mood is a significant part of the total disturbance.

yes ↓

no → Go to **C16**, page 35

C4

C. Continuous signs of the disturbance persist for at least 6 months. This 6-month period must include at least 1 month of symptoms (or less if successfully treated) that meet criterion A (i.e., active-phase symptoms) and may include periods of prodromal or residual symptoms. During these prodromal or residual periods, the signs of the disturbance may be manifested by only negative symptoms (i.e., affective flattening, alogia, avolition) or two or more symptoms listed in criterion A present in an attenuated form (e.g., odd beliefs, unusual perceptual experiences).

Question for clarification: Between [MULTIPLE EPISODES], were you back to your normal self? How long did each episode last?

yes ↓

no → Go to **C13**, page 34

C5

B. For a significant portion of the time since the onset of the disturbance, one or more major areas of functioning such as work, interpersonal relations, or self-care are markedly below the level achieved prior to the onset (or when the onset is in childhood or adolescence, failure to achieve expected level of interpersonal, academic, or occupational achievement).

Question for clarification: When you [had "A" CRITERION SYMPTOMS], were you having trouble working or taking care of yourself?

yes ↓

no → Go to **C39**, page 43

C6

E. The disturbance is not due to the direct physiological effects of a substance (e.g., a drug of abuse, a medication) or a general medical condition.

Questions for clarification: Were you taking any drugs or medicines during this time? Were you physically ill at this time?

If there is any indication that the psychotic symptoms may be secondary (i.e., a direct physiological consequence of a general medical condition or substance), go to page 39 and return here to make a rating of "yes" or "no."

Etiological general medical conditions include neurological conditions (e.g., neoplasms, cerebrovascular disease, Huntington's disease, epilepsy, auditory nerve injury, deafness, migraine, central nervous system infections), endocrine conditions (e.g., hyper- and hypothyroidism, hyper- and hypoparathyroidism, hypocortisolism), metabolic conditions (e.g., hypoxia, hypercarbia, hypoglycemia), fluid or electrolyte imbalances, hepatic or renal diseases, and autoimmune disorders with central nervous system involvement (e.g., systemic lupus erythematosis).

Etiological substances include alcohol, amphetamine, cannabis, cocaine, hallucinogens, inhalants, opioids (meperidine), phencyclidine, sedatives, hypnotics, anxiolytics, and other or unknown substances.

C6

yes (i.e., not due to a substance or general medical condition)

no → Go back to **C2,** page 29, if there are other psychotic symptoms not due to a substance or general medical condition; otherwise, go to **Module D**, page 45

C7

CRITERIA A, B, C, D, AND E ARE MET (MAKE A DIAGNOSIS OF SCHIZOPHRENIA). IF UNKNOWN: Have you had [PSYCHOTIC OR OTHER SYMPTOMS CODED "+"] in the past month?

C7

C8

Consider Paranoid Type: Currently (or most recently):

A. Preoccupation with one or more delusions or frequent auditory hallucinations.

B. None of the following is prominent: disorganized speech, disorganized or catatonic behavior, or flat or inappropriate affect.

C8

no

yes

295.30 Schizophrenia, Paranoid Type

Go to **Module D**, page 45

C9

Consider Catatonic Type: Currently (or most recently) the clinical picture is dominated by at least two of the following:

(1) motoric immobility as evidenced by catalepsy (including waxy flexibility) or stupor

(2) excessive motor activity (that is apparently purposeless and not influenced by external stimuli)

(3) extreme negativism (an apparently motiveless resistance to all instructions or maintenance of a rigid posture against attempts to be moved) or mutism

(4) peculiarities of voluntary movement as evidenced by posturing (voluntary assumption of inappropriate or bizarre postures), stereotyped movements, prominent mannerisms, or prominent grimacing

(5) echolalia or echopraxia

C9

no

yes

295.20 Schizophrenia, Catatonic Type

Go to **Module D**, page 45

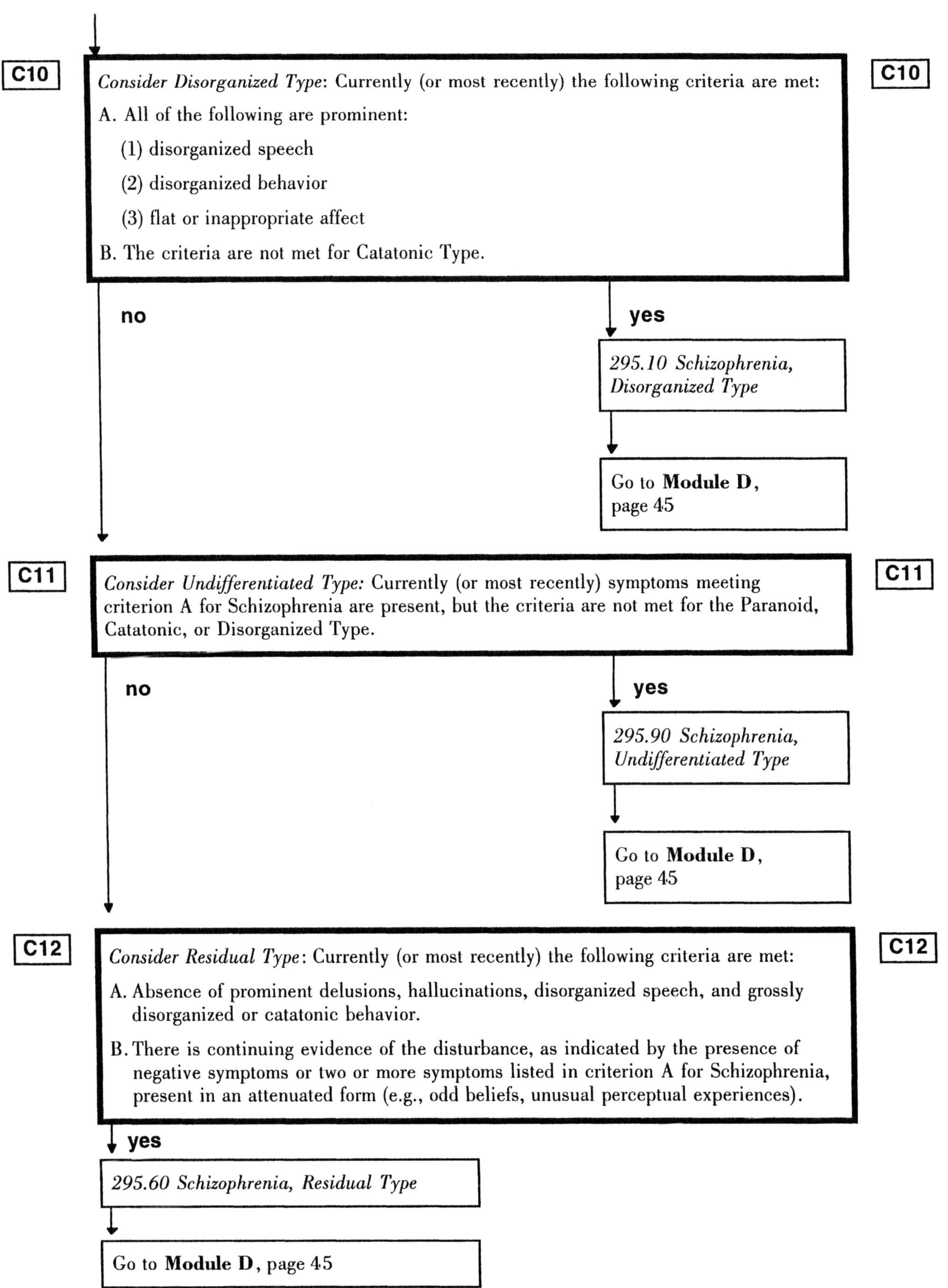

C10

Consider Disorganized Type: Currently (or most recently) the following criteria are met:

A. All of the following are prominent:

(1) disorganized speech

(2) disorganized behavior

(3) flat or inappropriate affect

B. The criteria are not met for Catatonic Type.

C10

no → C11

yes → *295.10 Schizophrenia, Disorganized Type* → Go to **Module D**, page 45

C11

Consider Undifferentiated Type: Currently (or most recently) symptoms meeting criterion A for Schizophrenia are present, but the criteria are not met for the Paranoid, Catatonic, or Disorganized Type.

C11

no → C12

yes → *295.90 Schizophrenia, Undifferentiated Type* → Go to **Module D**, page 45

C12

Consider Residual Type: Currently (or most recently) the following criteria are met:

A. Absence of prominent delusions, hallucinations, disorganized speech, and grossly disorganized or catatonic behavior.

B. There is continuing evidence of the disturbance, as indicated by the presence of negative symptoms or two or more symptoms listed in criterion A for Schizophrenia, present in an attenuated form (e.g., odd beliefs, unusual perceptual experiences).

C12

yes → *295.60 Schizophrenia, Residual Type* → Go to **Module D**, page 45

CRITERIA FOR SCHIZOPHRENIFORM DISORDER

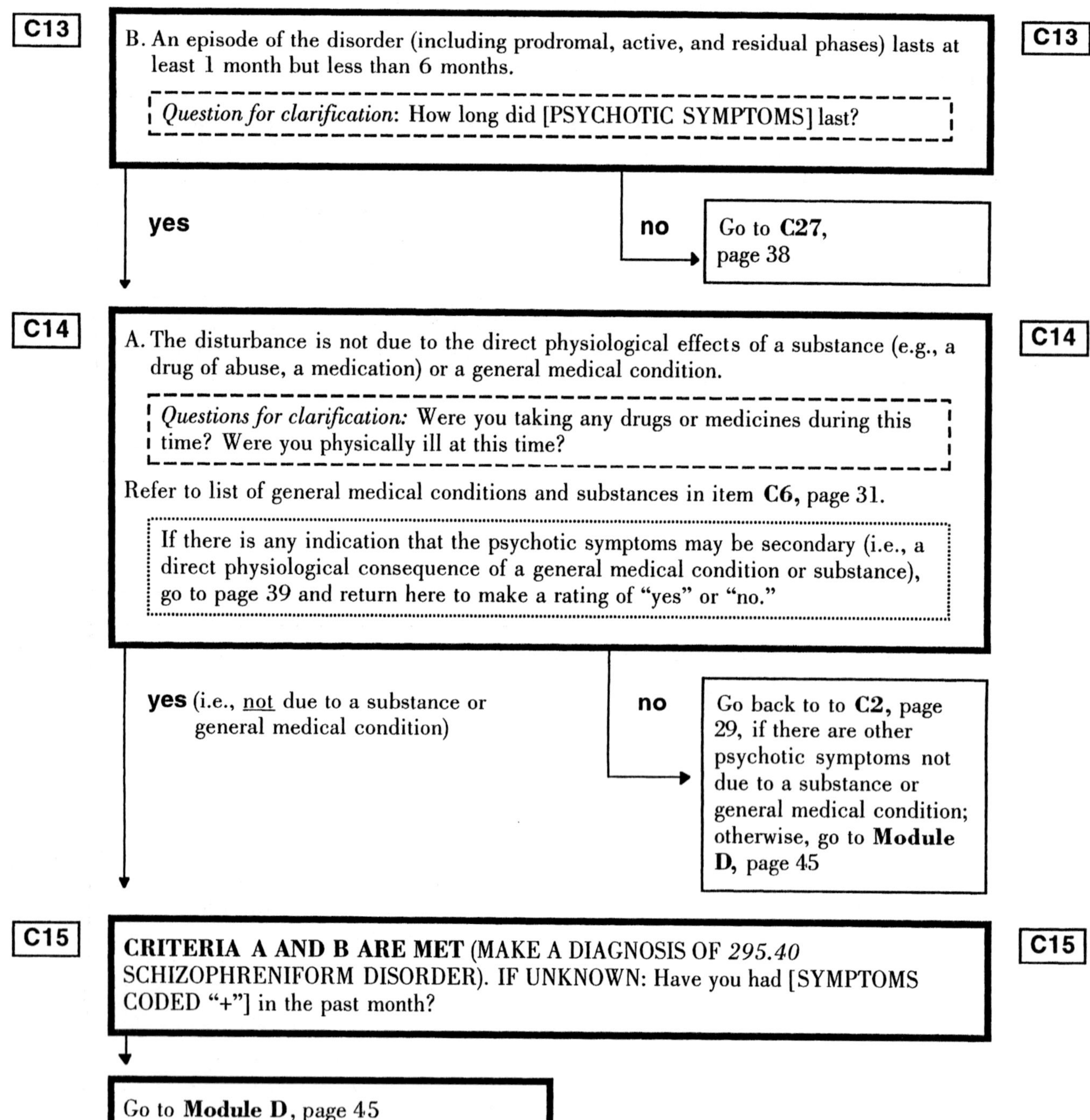

C13

B. An episode of the disorder (including prodromal, active, and residual phases) lasts at least 1 month but less than 6 months.

Question for clarification: How long did [PSYCHOTIC SYMPTOMS] last?

yes

no → Go to **C27**, page 38

C13

C14

A. The disturbance is not due to the direct physiological effects of a substance (e.g., a drug of abuse, a medication) or a general medical condition.

Questions for clarification: Were you taking any drugs or medicines during this time? Were you physically ill at this time?

Refer to list of general medical conditions and substances in item **C6,** page 31.

If there is any indication that the psychotic symptoms may be secondary (i.e., a direct physiological consequence of a general medical condition or substance), go to page 39 and return here to make a rating of "yes" or "no."

yes (i.e., not due to a substance or general medical condition)

no → Go back to to **C2,** page 29, if there are other psychotic symptoms not due to a substance or general medical condition; otherwise, go to **Module D,** page 45

C14

C15

CRITERIA A AND B ARE MET (MAKE A DIAGNOSIS OF *295.40* SCHIZOPHRENIFORM DISORDER). IF UNKNOWN: Have you had [SYMPTOMS CODED "+"] in the past month?

C15

Go to **Module D**, page 45

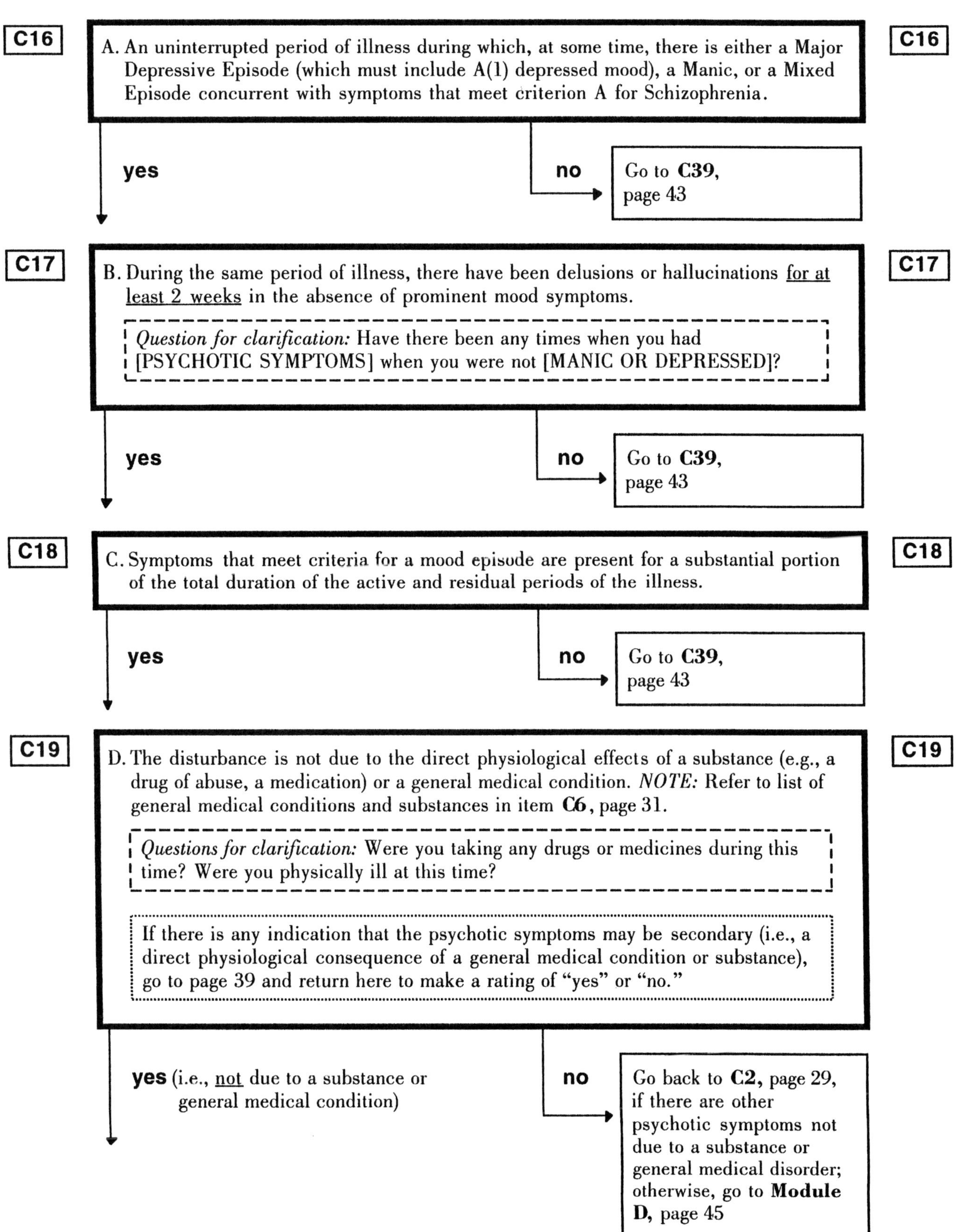

CRITERIA FOR SCHIZOAFFECTIVE DISORDER

C16 A. An uninterrupted period of illness during which, at some time, there is either a Major Depressive Episode (which must include A(1) depressed mood), a Manic, or a Mixed Episode concurrent with symptoms that meet criterion A for Schizophrenia. **C16**

yes ↓

no → Go to **C39**, page 43

C17 B. During the same period of illness, there have been delusions or hallucinations <u>for at least 2 weeks</u> in the absence of prominent mood symptoms. **C17**

Question for clarification: Have there been any times when you had [PSYCHOTIC SYMPTOMS] when you were not [MANIC OR DEPRESSED]?

yes ↓

no → Go to **C39**, page 43

C18 C. Symptoms that meet criteria for a mood episode are present for a substantial portion of the total duration of the active and residual periods of the illness. **C18**

yes ↓

no → Go to **C39**, page 43

C19 D. The disturbance is not due to the direct physiological effects of a substance (e.g., a drug of abuse, a medication) or a general medical condition. *NOTE:* Refer to list of general medical conditions and substances in item **C6**, page 31. **C19**

Questions for clarification: Were you taking any drugs or medicines during this time? Were you physically ill at this time?

If there is any indication that the psychotic symptoms may be secondary (i.e., a direct physiological consequence of a general medical condition or substance), go to page 39 and return here to make a rating of "yes" or "no."

yes (i.e., <u>not</u> due to a substance or general medical condition) ↓

no → Go back to **C2,** page 29, if there are other psychotic symptoms not due to a substance or general medical disorder; otherwise, go to **Module D,** page 45

C20 **CRITERIA A, B, C, AND D ARE MET** (MAKE A DIAGNOSIS OF *295.70* SCHIZOAFFECTIVE DISORDER). IF UNKNOWN: Have you had [SYMPTOMS CODED "+"] in the past month? C20

Go to **Module D**, page 45

CRITERIA FOR DELUSIONAL DISORDER

C21 A. Nonbizarre delusions (i.e., involving situations that occur in real life, such as being followed, poisoned, infected, loved at a distance, or deceived by a spouse or lover, or having a disease) of at least 1 month's duration. C21

yes

no → Go to **C27**, page 38

C22 B. Criterion A for Schizophrenia has never been met. **Note:** Tactile and olfactory hallucinations may be present in Delusional Disorder if they are related to the delusional theme. C22

yes

no → Go to **C39**, page 43

C23 C. Apart from the impact of the delusion(s) or its ramifications, functioning is not markedly impaired and behavior is not obviously odd or bizarre. C23

yes

no → Go to **C39**, page 43

C24 D. If mood episodes have occurred concurrently with delusions, their total duration has been brief relative to the duration of the delusional periods. C24

Questions for clarification: Has there ever been a time when you have believed [DELUSIONS] at the same time you were [depressed/high/irritable/OWN WORDS]? How much of the time that you have believed [DELUSIONS] would you say you have also been [depressed/high/irritable/OWN WORDS]?

NOTE: Answer "yes" if 1) there have never been any mood episodes at all, 2) mood episodes occurred at times other than during delusional periods, or 3) mood episodes were brief relative to total duration of the delusional periods. Answer "no" if symptoms meeting criteria for mood episodes have been present for a substantial portion of the total duration of the disturbance.

yes

no → Go to **C39**, page 43

C25

E. The disturbance is not due to the direct physiological effects of a substance (e.g., a drug of abuse, a medication) or a general medical condition. *NOTE:* Refer to list of general medical conditions and substances in item **C6**, page 31.

Questions for clarification: Were you taking any drugs or medicines during this time? Were you physically ill at this time?

If there is any indication that the psychotic symptoms may be secondary (i.e., a direct physiological consequence of a general medical condition or substance), go to page 39 and return here to make a rating of "yes" or "no."

C25

yes (i.e., not due to a substance or general medical condition)

no → Go back to **C2,** page 29, if there are other psychotic symptoms not due to a substance or general medical condition; otherwise, go to **Module D**, page 45

C26

CRITERIA A, B, C, D, AND E ARE MET (MAKE A DIAGNOSIS OF *297.1* DELUSIONAL DISORDER). IF UNKNOWN: Have you had [SYMPTOMS CODED "+"] in the past month?

C26

Go to **Module D**, page 45

CRITERIA FOR BRIEF PSYCHOTIC DISORDER

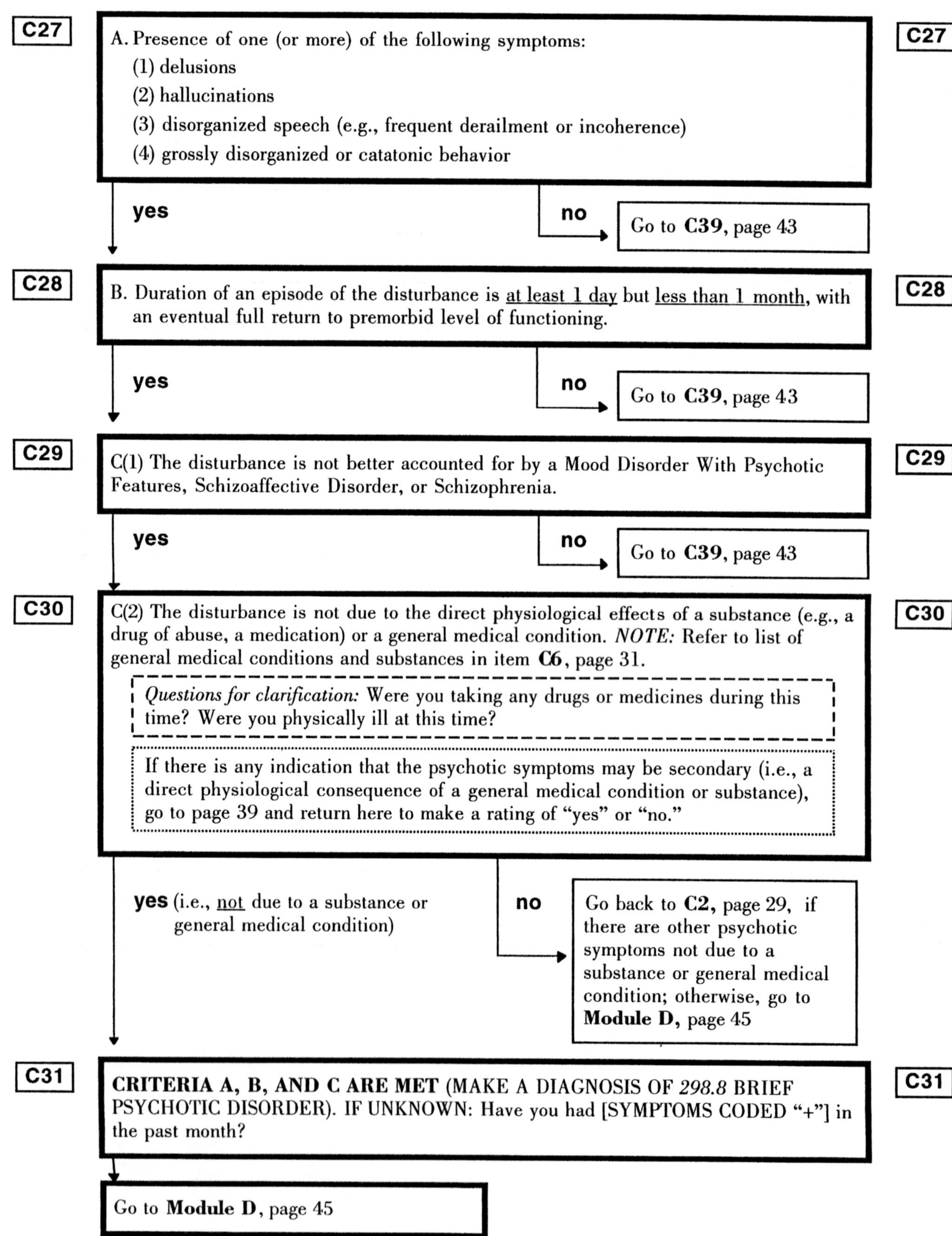

C27 A. Presence of one (or more) of the following symptoms:
(1) delusions
(2) hallucinations
(3) disorganized speech (e.g., frequent derailment or incoherence)
(4) grossly disorganized or catatonic behavior
C27

yes ↓ **no** → Go to **C39**, page 43

C28 B. Duration of an episode of the disturbance is <u>at least 1 day</u> but <u>less than 1 month</u>, with an eventual full return to premorbid level of functioning. **C28**

yes ↓ **no** → Go to **C39**, page 43

C29 C(1) The disturbance is not better accounted for by a Mood Disorder With Psychotic Features, Schizoaffective Disorder, or Schizophrenia. **C29**

yes ↓ **no** → Go to **C39**, page 43

C30 C(2) The disturbance is not due to the direct physiological effects of a substance (e.g., a drug of abuse, a medication) or a general medical condition. *NOTE:* Refer to list of general medical conditions and substances in item **C6**, page 31. **C30**

Questions for clarification: Were you taking any drugs or medicines during this time? Were you physically ill at this time?

If there is any indication that the psychotic symptoms may be secondary (i.e., a direct physiological consequence of a general medical condition or substance), go to page 39 and return here to make a rating of "yes" or "no."

yes (i.e., <u>not</u> due to a substance or general medical condition) ↓

no → Go back to **C2,** page 29, if there are other psychotic symptoms not due to a substance or general medical condition; otherwise, go to **Module D,** page 45

C31 **CRITERIA A, B, AND C ARE MET** (MAKE A DIAGNOSIS OF *298.8* BRIEF PSYCHOTIC DISORDER). IF UNKNOWN: Have you had [SYMPTOMS CODED "+"] in the past month? **C31**

Go to **Module D**, page 45

CONSIDER ETIOLOGICAL ROLE OF A GENERAL MEDICAL CONDITION OR SUBSTANCE USE

If psychotic symptoms are <u>not</u> temporally associated with a general medical condition, go to **C35**, page 41 (*Substance-Induced Psychotic Disorder*).

PSYCHOTIC DISORDER DUE TO A GENERAL MEDICAL CONDITION	CRITERIA FOR PSYCHOTIC DISORDER DUE TO A GENERAL MEDICAL CONDITION	
	NOTE: Criterion D (i.e., not during delirium) has been omitted from the SCID.	
C32 CODE BASED ON INFORMATION ALREADY OBTAINED	A. Prominent hallucinations or delusions.	**C32**
C33 Do you think your [DELUSIONS/ HALLUCINATIONS] were in any way related to your [COMORBID GENERAL MEDICAL CONDITION]? IF YES: Tell me how. (Did the [DELUSIONS/ HALLUCINATIONS] start or get much worse only after [COMORBID GENERAL MEDICAL CONDITION] began?) IF YES AND GENERAL MEDICAL CONDITION HAS RESOLVED: Did the [DELUSIONS/HALLUCINATIONS] get better once the [COMORBID GENERAL MEDICAL CONDITION] got better?	B/C. There is evidence from the history, physical examination, or laboratory findings that the disturbance is the direct physiological consequence of a general medical condition, and the disturbance is not better accounted for by another mental disorder.	**C33**

If **C33** is "–" (general medical condition not etiological), go to **C35**, page 41 (*Substance-Induced Psychotic Disorder*).

C34	IF UNKNOWN: Have you had [SYMPTOMS CODED "+"] in the past month?	**CRITERIA A AND B/C ARE MET** (MAKE A DIAGNOSIS OF PSYCHOTIC DISORDER DUE TO A GENERAL MEDICAL CONDITION)	C34

If psychotic symptoms are not temporally associated with substance use, return to disorder being evaluated:

C6 for Schizophrenia (page 31)

C14 for Schizophreniform Disorder (page 34)

C19 for Schizoaffective Disorder (page 35)

C25 for Delusional Disorder (page 37)

C30 for Brief Psychotic Disorder (page 38)

SUBSTANCE-INDUCED PSYCHOTIC DISORDER

CRITERIA FOR SUBSTANCE-INDUCED PSYCHOTIC DISORDER

NOTE: Criterion D (i.e., not during delirium) has been omitted from the SCID.

C35 CODE BASED ON INFORMATION ALREADY OBTAINED

A. Prominent hallucinations or delusions. **Note:** Do not include hallucinations if the person has insight (while they are experienced) that they are substance induced. **C35**

C36 IF NOT KNOWN: When did the [DELUSIONS/HALLUCINATIONS] begin? Were you already using [SUBSTANCE] or had you just stopped or cut down your use?

B. There is evidence from the history, physical examination, or laboratory findings of either (1) or (2) **C36**

(1) the symptoms in criterion A developed during, or within a month of, Substance Intoxication or Withdrawal

(2) medication use is etiologically related to the disturbance.

If **C36** is "–" (i.e., not etiologically related to a substance), return to disorder being evaluated:

C6 for Schizophrenia (page 31)

C14 for Schizophreniform Disorder (page 34)

C19 for Schizoaffective Disorder (page 35)

C25 for Delusional Disorder (page 37)

C30 for Brief Psychotic Disorder (page 38)

C37 Do you think your [DELUSIONS/HALLUCINATIONS] are in any way related to your [SUBSTANCE USE]?

IF YES: Tell me how.

ASK ANY OF THE FOLLOWING QUESTIONS AS NEEDED TO RULE OUT A NONSUBSTANCE ETIOLOGY

IF UNKNOWN: Which came first, the [SUBSTANCE USE] or the [DELUSIONS/HALLUCINATIONS]?

C. The disturbance is not better accounted for by a Psychotic Disorder that is not substance induced. Evidence that the symptoms are better accounted for by a Psychotic Disorder that is not substance induced might include: **C37**

(1) the psychotic symptoms precede the onset of the substance use (or medication use)

C37 (cont'd)

IF UNKNOWN: Have you had a period of time when you stopped using [SUBSTANCE]?

IF YES: After you stopped using [SUBSTANCE] did the [DELUSIONS/ HALLUCINATIONS] get better?

(2) the psychotic symptoms persist for a substantial period of time (e.g., about a month) after the cessation of acute withdrawal or severe intoxication

IF UNKNOWN: How much of [SUBSTANCE] were you using when you began to have [DELUSIONS/ HALLUCINATIONS]?

(3) the psychotic symptoms are substantially in excess of what would be expected given the type or amount of the substance used or the duration of use

IF UNKNOWN: Have you had any other episodes of [DELUSIONS/ HALLUCINATIONS]?

IF YES: How many? Were you using [SUBSTANCE] at those times?

(4) there is other evidence that suggests the existence of an independent non-substance-induced Psychotic Disorder (e.g., a history of recurrent non-substance-related psychotic episodes).

C37 (cont'd)

If **C37** is "–" (i.e., the disturbance is better accounted for by a non-substance-induced psychotic disorder), return to disorder being evaluated:

C6 for Schizophrenia (page 31)

C14 for Schizophreniform Disorder (page 34)

C19 for Schizoaffective Disorder (page 35)

C25 for Delusional Disorder (page 37)

C30 for Brief Psychotic Disorder (page 38)

C38

IF UNKNOWN: Have you had [SYMPTOMS CODED "+"] in the past month?

CRITERIA A, B, AND C ARE MET
(MAKE A DIAGNOSIS OF SUBSTANCE-INDUCED PSYCHOTIC DISORDER)

C38

Return to disorder being evaluated:

C6 for Schizophrenia (page 31)

C14 for Schizophreniform Disorder (page 34)

C19 for Schizoaffective Disorder (page 35)

C25 for Delusional Disorder (page 37)

C30 for Brief Psychotic Disorder (page 38)

298.9 PSYCHOTIC DISORDER NOT OTHERWISE SPECIFIED

C39

This category should be used to diagnose psychotic symptomatology (i.e., delusions, hallucinations, disorganized speech, grossly disorganized or catatonic behavior) about which there is inadequate information to make a specific diagnosis or about which there is contradictory information, or disorders with psychotic symptoms that do not meet the criteria for any specific Psychotic Disorder defined above.

IF UNKNOWN: Have you had [PSYCHOTIC SYMPTOMS] in the past month?

C39

Go to **Module D**, page 45

D. MOOD DISORDERS

If there have never been any clinically significant mood symptoms, or if all mood symptoms are accounted for by a diagnosis of Schizoaffective Disorder (see **Module C,** page 29), go to **Module E,** page 53.

CRITERIA FOR BIPOLAR I DISORDER

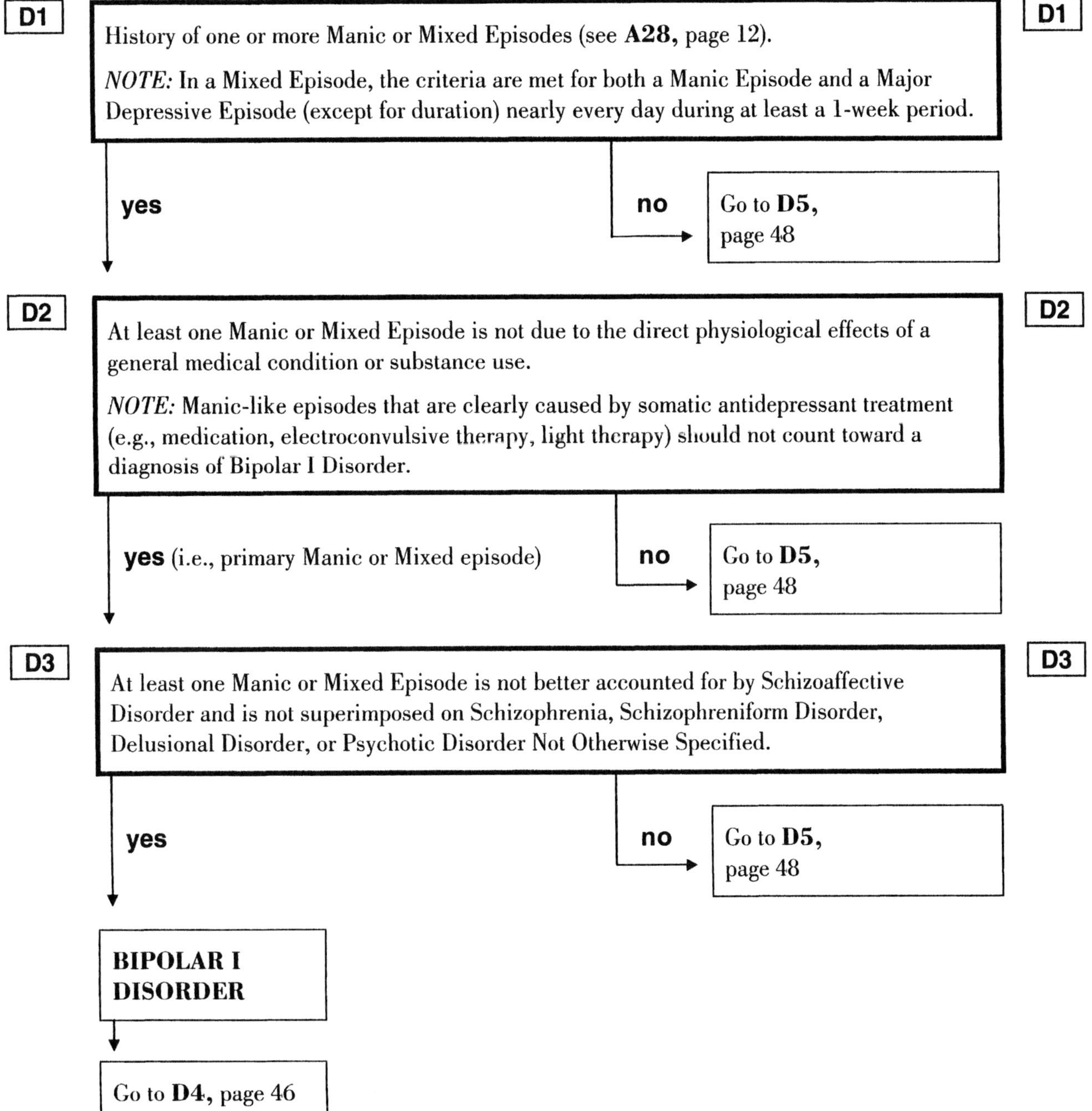

D1 — History of one or more Manic or Mixed Episodes (see **A28,** page 12).

NOTE: In a Mixed Episode, the criteria are met for both a Manic Episode and a Major Depressive Episode (except for duration) nearly every day during at least a 1-week period. — D1

yes ↓ **no** → Go to **D5,** page 48

D2 — At least one Manic or Mixed Episode is not due to the direct physiological effects of a general medical condition or substance use.

NOTE: Manic-like episodes that are clearly caused by somatic antidepressant treatment (e.g., medication, electroconvulsive therapy, light therapy) should not count toward a diagnosis of Bipolar I Disorder. — D2

yes (i.e., primary Manic or Mixed episode) ↓ **no** → Go to **D5,** page 48

D3 — At least one Manic or Mixed Episode is not better accounted for by Schizoaffective Disorder and is not superimposed on Schizophrenia, Schizophreniform Disorder, Delusional Disorder, or Psychotic Disorder Not Otherwise Specified. — D3

yes ↓ **no** → Go to **D5,** page 48

BIPOLAR I DISORDER

↓

Go to **D4,** page 46

D4

Select diagnostic code based on current (or most recent) episode (fifth digit is based on severity):

IF UNKNOWN: Have you had [MANIC OR DEPRESSIVE SYMPTOMS] in the past month?

296.40 Bipolar I Disorder, Most Recent Episode Hypomanic

296.0x Bipolar I Disorder, Single Manic Episode
296.4x Bipolar I Disorder, Most Recent Episode Manic

1—**Mild:** Minimum symptom criteria are met for a Manic Episode.
2—**Moderate:** Extreme increase in activity or impairment in judgment.
3—**Severe Without Psychotic Features:** Almost continual supervision required to prevent physical harm to self or others.
4—**Severe With Psychotic Features:** Delusions or hallucinations. If possible, specify whether psychotic features are mood-congruent or mood-incongruent:
Mood-Congruent Psychotic Features: Delusions or hallucinations whose content is entirely consistent with the typical manic themes of inflated worth, power, knowledge, identity, or special relationship to a deity or famous person.
Mood-Incongruent Psychotic Features: Delusions or hallucinations whose content does not involve typical manic themes of inflated worth, power, knowledge, identity, or special relationship to a deity or famous person. Included are symptoms such as persecutory delusions (not directly related to grandiose ideas or themes), thought insertion, and delusions of being controlled.
5—**In Partial Remission:** Symptoms of a Manic Episode are present but full criteria are not met, or there is a period without any significant symptoms of a Manic Episode lasting less than 2 months, following the end of the Manic Episode.
6—**In Full Remission:** During the past 2 months, no significant signs or symptoms of the disturbance were present.
0—**Unspecified.**

296.6x Bipolar I Disorder, Most Recent Episode Mixed

1—**Mild:** No more than minimum symptom criteria are met for both a Manic Episode and a Major Depressive Episode.
2—**Moderate:** Symptoms or functional impairment between "mild" and "severe."
3—**Severe Without Psychotic Features:** Almost continual supervision required to prevent physical harm to self or others.
4—**Severe With Psychotic Features:** Delusions or hallucinations. If possible, specify whether psychotic features are mood-congruent or mood-incongruent:
Mood-Congruent Psychotic Features: Delusions or hallucinations whose content is entirely consistent with the typical manic or depressive themes.
Mood-Incongruent Psychotic Features: Delusions or hallucinations whose content does not involve typical manic or depressive themes. Included are symptoms such as persecutory delusions (not directly related to grandiose or depressive themes), thought insertion, and delusions of being controlled.
5—**In Partial Remission:** Symptoms of a Mixed Episode are present but full criteria are not met, or there is a period without any significant symptoms of a Mixed Episode lasting less than 2 months following the end of the Mixed Episode.
6—**In Full Remission:** During the past 2 months, no significant signs or symptoms of the disturbance were present.
0—**Unspecified.**

D4

D4 (cont'd)

296.5x Bipolar I Disorder, Most Recent Episode Depressed

1—**Mild:** Few, if any, symptoms in excess of those required to make the diagnosis, and symptoms result in only minor impairment in occupational functioning or in usual social activities or relationships with others.

2—**Moderate:** Symptoms or functional impairment between "mild" and "severe."

3—**Severe Without Psychotic Features:** Several symptoms in excess of those required to make the diagnosis, and symptoms markedly interfere with occupational functioning or with usual social activities or relationships with others.

4—**Severe With Psychotic Features:** Delusions or hallucinations. If possible, specify whether psychotic features are mood-congruent or mood-incongruent:

Mood-Congruent Psychotic Features: Delusions or hallucinations whose content is entirely consistent with the typical depressive themes of personal inadequacy, guilt, disease, death, nihilism, or deserved punishment.

Mood-Incongruent Psychotic Features: Delusions or hallucinations whose content does not involve typical depressive themes of personal inadequacy, guilt, disease, death, nihilism, or deserved punishment. Included are symptoms such as persecutory delusions (not directly related to grandiose or depressive themes), thought insertion, thought broadcasting, and delusions of control.

5—**In Partial Remission:** Symptoms of a Major Depressive Episode are present but full criteria are not met, or there is a period without any significant symptoms of a Major Depressive Episode lasting less than 2 months following the end of the Major Depressive Episode. (If the Major Depressive Episode was superimposed on Dysthymic Disorder, the diagnosis of Dysthymic Disorder alone is given once the full criteria for a Major Depressive Episode are no longer met.)

6—**In Full Remission:** During the past 2 months, no significant signs or symptoms of the disturbance were present.

0—**Unspecified.**

296.7 Bipolar I Disorder, Most Recent Episode Unspecified (Criteria, except for duration, are currently [or most recently] met for a Manic, a Hypomanic, a Mixed, or a Major Depressive Episode.)

D4 (cont'd)

Go to **Module E**, page 53

CRITERIA FOR BIPOLAR II DISORDER

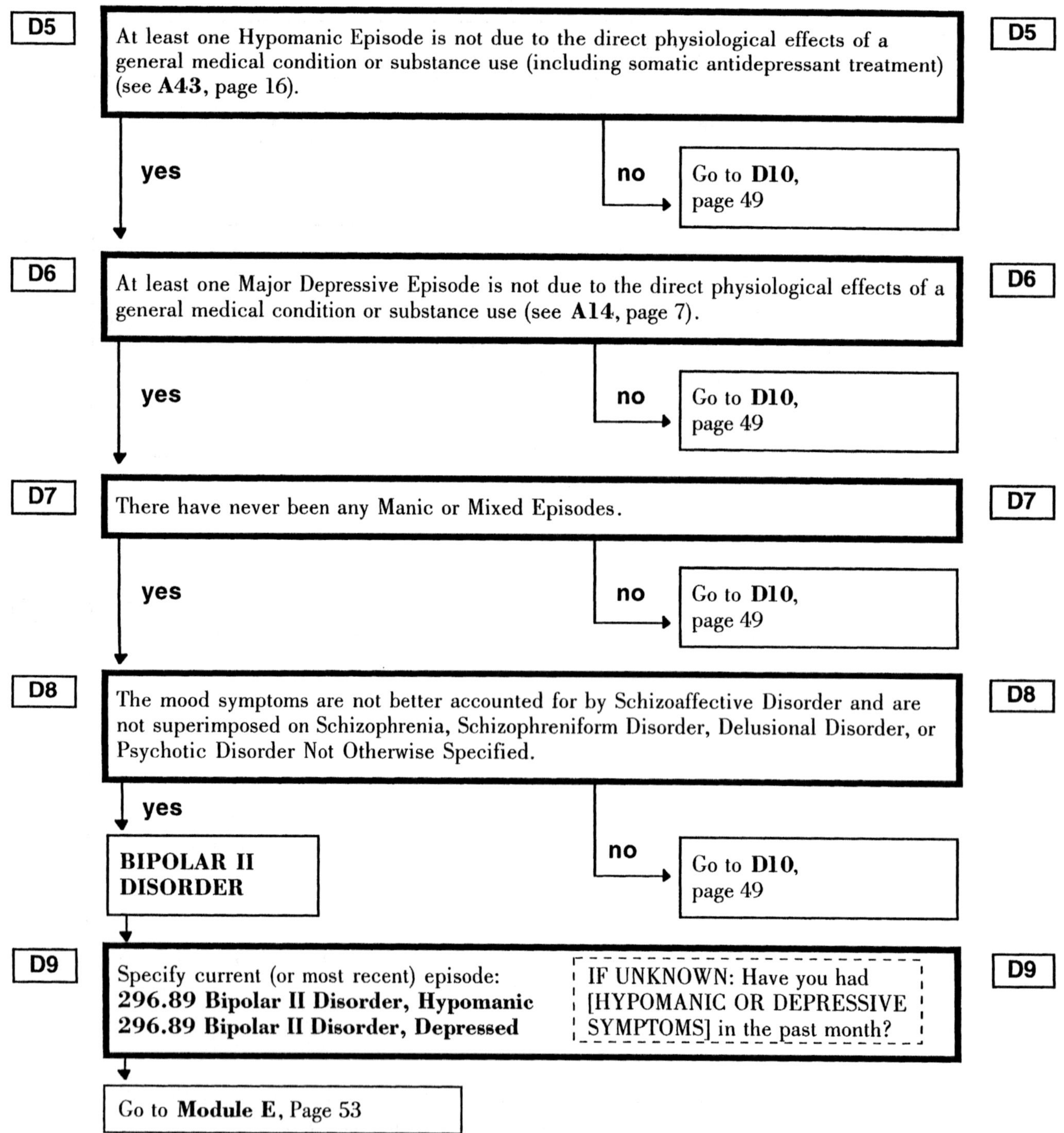

D5 At least one Hypomanic Episode is not due to the direct physiological effects of a general medical condition or substance use (including somatic antidepressant treatment) (see **A43**, page 16). **D5**

yes ↓

no → Go to **D10**, page 49

D6 At least one Major Depressive Episode is not due to the direct physiological effects of a general medical condition or substance use (see **A14**, page 7). **D6**

yes ↓

no → Go to **D10**, page 49

D7 There have never been any Manic or Mixed Episodes. **D7**

yes ↓

no → Go to **D10**, page 49

D8 The mood symptoms are not better accounted for by Schizoaffective Disorder and are not superimposed on Schizophrenia, Schizophreniform Disorder, Delusional Disorder, or Psychotic Disorder Not Otherwise Specified. **D8**

yes ↓

BIPOLAR II DISORDER

no → Go to **D10**, page 49

D9 Specify current (or most recent) episode:
296.89 Bipolar II Disorder, Hypomanic
296.89 Bipolar II Disorder, Depressed

IF UNKNOWN: Have you had [HYPOMANIC OR DEPRESSIVE SYMPTOMS] in the past month? **D9**

↓

Go to **Module E**, Page 53

OTHER BIPOLAR DISORDERS

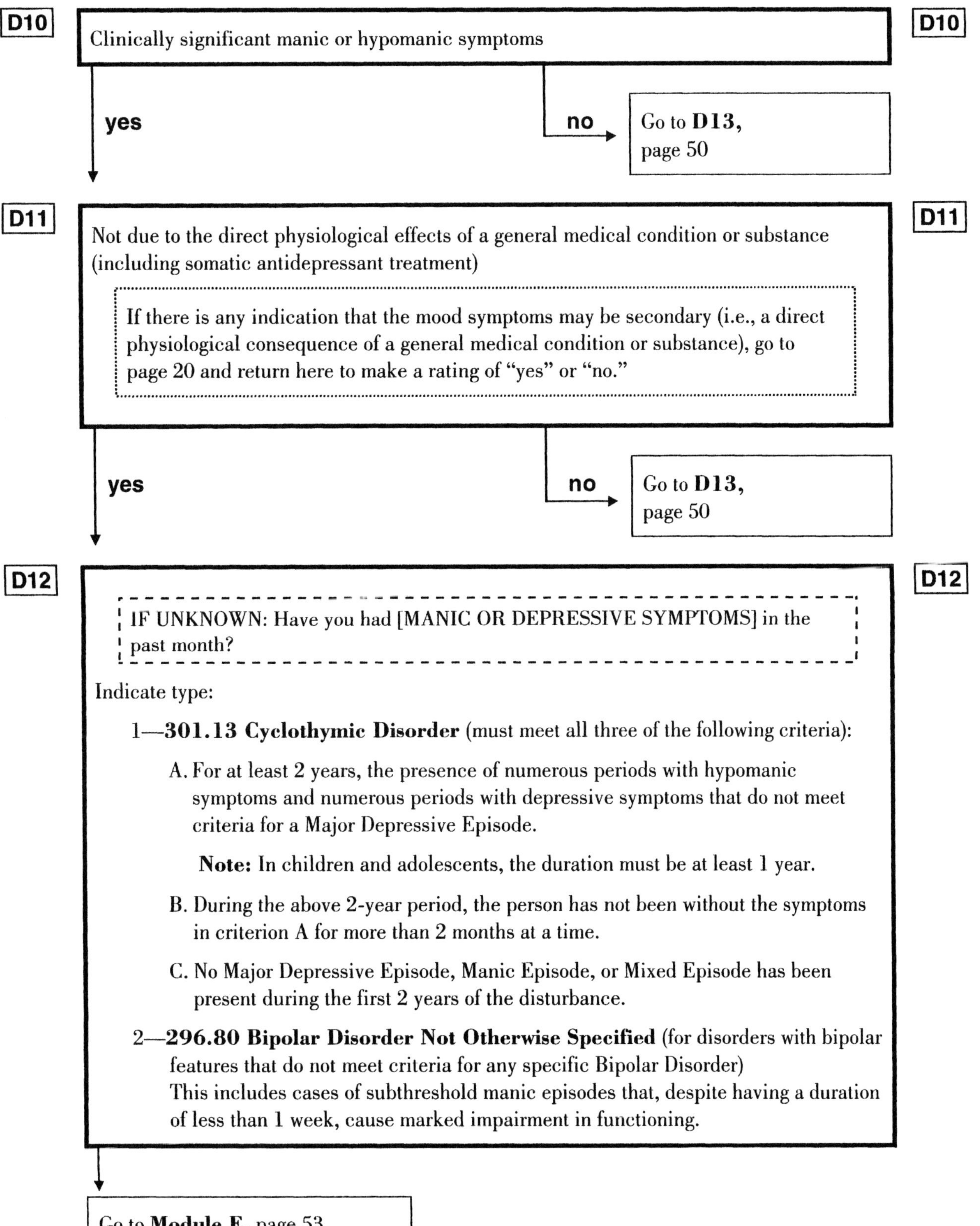

D10 Clinically significant manic or hypomanic symptoms D10

yes ↓

no → Go to **D13,** page 50

D11 Not due to the direct physiological effects of a general medical condition or substance (including somatic antidepressant treatment) D11

If there is any indication that the mood symptoms may be secondary (i.e., a direct physiological consequence of a general medical condition or substance), go to page 20 and return here to make a rating of "yes" or "no."

yes ↓

no → Go to **D13,** page 50

D12 D12

IF UNKNOWN: Have you had [MANIC OR DEPRESSIVE SYMPTOMS] in the past month?

Indicate type:

1—**301.13 Cyclothymic Disorder** (must meet all three of the following criteria):

A. For at least 2 years, the presence of numerous periods with hypomanic symptoms and numerous periods with depressive symptoms that do not meet criteria for a Major Depressive Episode.

Note: In children and adolescents, the duration must be at least 1 year.

B. During the above 2-year period, the person has not been without the symptoms in criterion A for more than 2 months at a time.

C. No Major Depressive Episode, Manic Episode, or Mixed Episode has been present during the first 2 years of the disturbance.

2—**296.80 Bipolar Disorder Not Otherwise Specified** (for disorders with bipolar features that do not meet criteria for any specific Bipolar Disorder)
This includes cases of subthreshold manic episodes that, despite having a duration of less than 1 week, cause marked impairment in functioning.

↓

Go to **Module E,** page 53

CRITERIA FOR MAJOR DEPRESSIVE DISORDER

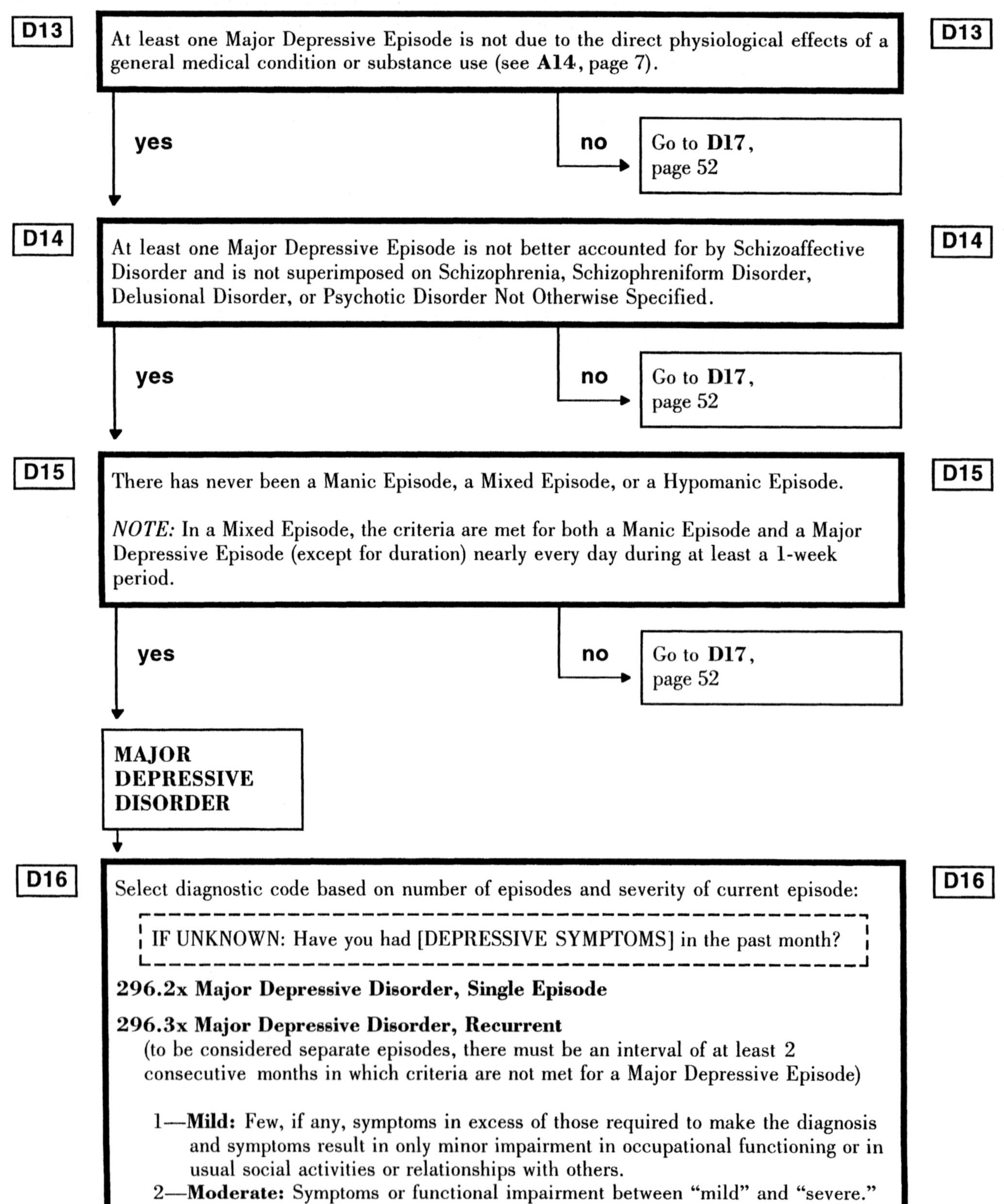

D13 At least one Major Depressive Episode is not due to the direct physiological effects of a general medical condition or substance use (see **A14**, page 7). **D13**

yes → (continue)

no → Go to **D17**, page 52

D14 At least one Major Depressive Episode is not better accounted for by Schizoaffective Disorder and is not superimposed on Schizophrenia, Schizophreniform Disorder, Delusional Disorder, or Psychotic Disorder Not Otherwise Specified. **D14**

yes → (continue)

no → Go to **D17**, page 52

D15 There has never been a Manic Episode, a Mixed Episode, or a Hypomanic Episode. **D15**

NOTE: In a Mixed Episode, the criteria are met for both a Manic Episode and a Major Depressive Episode (except for duration) nearly every day during at least a 1-week period.

yes → (continue)

no → Go to **D17**, page 52

MAJOR DEPRESSIVE DISORDER

D16 Select diagnostic code based on number of episodes and severity of current episode: **D16**

IF UNKNOWN: Have you had [DEPRESSIVE SYMPTOMS] in the past month?

296.2x Major Depressive Disorder, Single Episode

296.3x Major Depressive Disorder, Recurrent
(to be considered separate episodes, there must be an interval of at least 2 consecutive months in which criteria are not met for a Major Depressive Episode)

1—**Mild:** Few, if any, symptoms in excess of those required to make the diagnosis and symptoms result in only minor impairment in occupational functioning or in usual social activities or relationships with others.
2—**Moderate:** Symptoms or functional impairment between "mild" and "severe."

D16 (cont'd)

3—**Severe Without Psychotic Features:** Several symptoms in excess of those required to make the diagnosis and symptoms markedly interfere with occupational functioning or with usual social activities or relationships with others.

4—**Severe With Psychotic Features:** Delusions or hallucinations. If possible, specify whether psychotic features are mood-congruent or mood-incongruent:

Mood-Congruent Psychotic Features: Delusions or hallucinations whose content is entirely consistent with the typical depressive themes of personal inadequacy, guilt, disease, death, nihilism, or deserved punishment.

Mood-Incongruent Psychotic Features: Delusions or hallucinations whose content does not involve typical depressive themes of personal inadequacy, guilt, disease, death, nihilsm, or deserved punishment. Included are symptoms such as persecutory delusions (not directly related to grandiose or depressive themes), thought insertion, thought broadcasting, and delusions of control.

5—**In Partial Remission:** Symptoms of a Major Depressive Episode are present but full criteria are not met, or there is a period without any significant symptoms of a Major Depressive Episode lasting less than 2 months following the end of the Major Depressive Episode. (If the Major Depressive Episode was superimposed on Dysthymic Disorder, the diagnosis of Dysthymic Disorder alone is given once the full criteria for a Major Depressive Episode are no longer met.)

6—**In Full Remission:** During the past 2 months, no significant signs or symptoms of the disturbance were present.

0—**Unspecified.**

D16 (cont'd)

Go to **Module E**, page 53

DEPRESSIVE DISORDER NOT OTHERWISE SPECIFIED

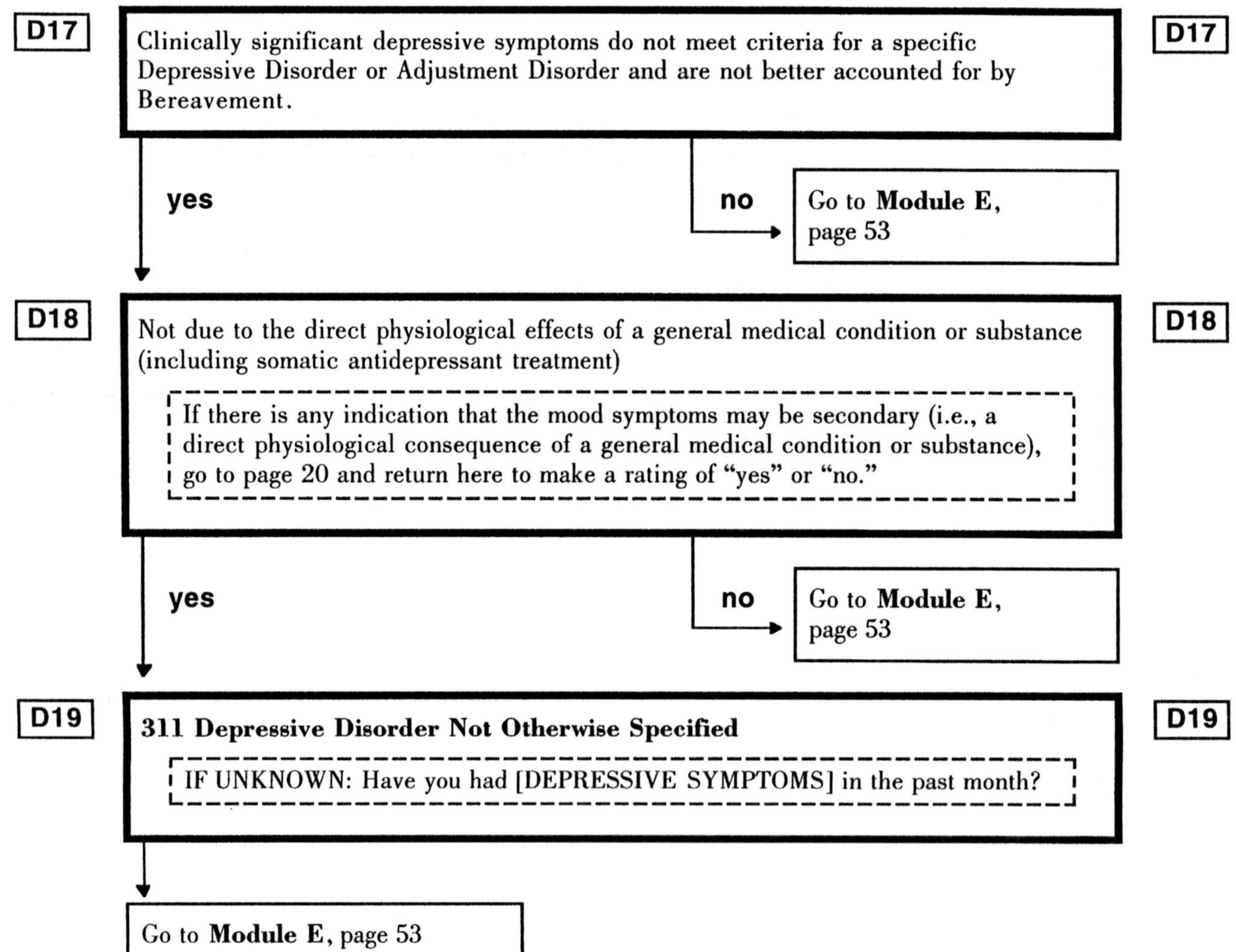

D17 Clinically significant depressive symptoms do not meet criteria for a specific Depressive Disorder or Adjustment Disorder and are not better accounted for by Bereavement. D17

yes

no — Go to **Module E,** page 53

D18 Not due to the direct physiological effects of a general medical condition or substance (including somatic antidepressant treatment) D18

If there is any indication that the mood symptoms may be secondary (i.e., a direct physiological consequence of a general medical condition or substance), go to page 20 and return here to make a rating of "yes" or "no."

yes

no — Go to **Module E,** page 53

D19 **311 Depressive Disorder Not Otherwise Specified** D19

IF UNKNOWN: Have you had [DEPRESSIVE SYMPTOMS] in the past month?

Go to **Module E,** page 53

E. ALCOHOL AND OTHER SUBSTANCE USE DISORDERS

What are your drinking habits like? (How much do you drink?) (How often?) (What do you drink?)

IF NOT CURRENTLY DRINKING HEAVILY: Was there ever a time in your life when you were drinking a lot more? (How often were you drinking?) (What were you drinking? How much? How long did that period last?)

(Currently/During that time . . .)

. . . (does/did) your drinking cause problems for you?

. . . (does/did) anyone object to your drinking?

If *Alcohol Dependence* seems likely, go to **E7** (page 55).

E1 has ever had a period of excessive drinking OR has ever had any evidence of alcohol-related problems **E1**

If **E1** is "–" (i.e., never excessive drinking AND never alcohol-related problems), go to **E17,** page 58 *(Nonalcohol Substance Use Disorders).*

ALCOHOL ABUSE

Let me ask you a few more questions about [TIME WHEN DRINKING MOST/TIME WITH MOST PROBLEMS]. During that time . . .

CRITERIA FOR ALCOHOL ABUSE

A. A maladaptive pattern of substance use leading to clinically significant impairment or distress as manifested by one (or more) of the following occurring within a 12-month period:

E2 Did you miss work or school because you were intoxicated, high, or very hung over? (How often? What about doing a bad job at work or failing courses at school because of your drinking?)

IF NO: What about not keeping your house clean or not taking proper care of your children because of your drinking? (How often?)

(1) recurrent alcohol use resulting in a failure to fulfill major role obligations at work, school, or home (e.g., repeated absences or poor work performance related to alcohol use; alcohol-related absences, suspensions, or expulsions from school; neglect of children or household) **E2**

E3	Did you ever drink in a situation in which it might have been dangerous to drink at all? (Did you ever drive while you were really too drunk to drive?) IF YES: How many times? (When?)	(2) recurrent alcohol use in situations in which it is physically hazardous (e.g., driving an automobile or operating a machine when impaired by alcohol use)	**E3**
E4	Did your drinking get you into trouble with the law? (Tell me more about that.) IF YES: How many times? (When?)	(3) recurrent alcohol-related legal problems (e.g., arrests for alcohol-related disorderly conduct)	**E4**
E5	IF NOT ALREADY KNOWN: Did your drinking cause problems with other people, such as with family members, friends, or people at work? (Did you ever get into physical fights when you were drinking? What about having bad arguments about your drinking?) IF YES: Did you keep on drinking anyway?	(4) continued alcohol use despite having persistent or recurrent social or interpersonal problems caused or exacerbated by the effects of alcohol (e.g., arguments with spouse about consequences of intoxication, physical fights)	**E5**
E6		**AT LEAST ONE ABUSE ITEM IS "+"**	**E6**

If **E6** is "–" (i.e., no abuse items are "+"), go to **E17,** page 58 *(Nonalcohol Substance Use Disorders).*

If **E6** is "+" (i.e., at least one abuse item is "+") AND you have already checked for Dependence (i.e., evaluated **E7–E13** on pages 55–56) and found that fewer than three were "+," go to **E16,** page 57, and make a diagnosis of *Alcohol Abuse.*

ALCOHOL DEPENDENCE

Now I would like to ask you some more questions about [TIME WHEN DRINKING THE MOST/TIME WHEN DRINKING CAUSED THE MOST PROBLEMS]. During that time . . .

CRITERIA FOR ALCOHOL DEPENDENCE

A maladaptive pattern of alcohol use, leading to clinically significant impairment or distress, as manifested by three (or more) of the following occurring at any time in the same 12-month period:

NOTE: Criteria for Dependence are presented in a different order than in DSM-IV.

E7 Did you often find that when you started drinking you ended up drinking much more than you were planning to?

IF NO: What about drinking over a much longer period of time than you were planning to?

(3) alcohol is often taken in larger amounts OR over a longer period than was intended **E7**

E8 Did you try to cut down or stop drinking alcohol?

IF YES: Did you ever actually stop drinking altogether? (How many times did you try to cut down or stop altogether?)

IF NO: Did you want to stop or cut down? (Is this something you kept worrying about?)

(4) there is a persistent desire OR unsuccessful efforts to cut down or control substance use **E8**

E9 Did you spend a lot of time drinking, being high, or hung over?

(5) a great deal of time is spent in activities necessary to obtain alcohol, use alcohol, or recover from its effects **E9**

E10 Did you often have times when you would drink so often that you started to drink instead of working, spending time with your family or friends, or engaging in other important activities, such as sports, gardening, or playing music?

(6) important social, occupational, or recreational activities are given up or reduced because of alcohol use **E10**

E11

IF NOT ALREADY KNOWN: Did your drinking cause any psychological problems such as making you depressed or anxious, making it hard to sleep, or causing "blackouts"?

IF NOT ALREADY KNOWN: Did your drinking cause significant physical problems or make a physical problem worse?

IF YES TO EITHER OF ABOVE: Did you keep on drinking anyway?

(7) alcohol use is continued despite knowledge of having a persistent or recurrent physical or psychological problem that is likely to have been caused or exacerbated by alcohol (e.g., continued drinking despite recognition that an ulcer was made worse by alcohol consumption) **E11**

E12

Did you find that you needed to drink a lot more in order to get the feeling you wanted than you did when you first started drinking?

IF YES: How much more?

IF NO: What about finding that when you drank the same amount, it had much less effect than before?

(1) tolerance, as defined by either of the following: **E12**

(a) a need for markedly increased amounts of alcohol to achieve intoxication or desired effect

(b) markedly diminished effect with continued use of the same amount of alcohol

E13

Did you ever have any withdrawal symptoms when you cut down or stopped drinking such as . . .
. . . sweating or racing heart?
. . . hand shakes?
. . . trouble sleeping?
. . . feeling nauseated or vomiting?
. . . feeling agitated?
. . . or feeling anxious?

(How about having a seizure or seeing, feeling, or hearing things that weren't really there?)

IF NO: Did you ever start the day with a drink, or did you often drink or take some other drug or medication to keep yourself from getting the shakes or becoming sick?

(2) withdrawal, as manifested by either (a) or (b): **E13**

(a) at least <u>two</u> of the following developing within several hours to a few days after cessation of (or reduction in) heavy and prolonged alcohol use:
—autonomic hyperactivity (e.g., sweating or pulse rate greater than 100)
—increased hand tremor
—insomnia
—nausea or vomiting
—psychomotor agitation
—anxiety
—grand mal seizures
—transient visual, tactile, or auditory hallucinations or illusions

(b) alcohol (or a substance from the sedative/hypnotic/anxiolytic class) taken to relieve or avoid withdrawal symptoms

E14	IF UNKNOWN: When did [SYMPTOMS RATED "+" ABOVE] occur? (Did they all happen around the same time?)	**AT LEAST THREE DEPENDENCE ITEMS (E7–E13) ARE "+" AND OCCURRED WITHIN THE SAME 12-MONTH PERIOD**	**E14**

If **E14** is "–" (fewer than three dependence items are "+") AND you previously skipped **E2–E5** (because dependence seemed likely), return to **E2**, page 53, and check for *Alcohol Abuse*.

If **E14** is "–" (fewer than three dependence items are "+") AND **E6**, page 54, is "+" (criteria met for *Alcohol Abuse*) go to **E16** (below).

E15	IF UNKNOWN: Have you had [SYMPTOMS RATED "+" ABOVE] in the past month?	**MAKE A DIAGNOSIS OF ALCOHOL DEPENDENCE**	**E15**

Go to **E17**, page 58 (*Nonalcohol Substance Use Disorders*).

E16	IF UNKNOWN: Have you had [SYMPTOMS OF ABUSE RATED "+"] in the past month?	**MAKE A DIAGNOSIS OF ALCOHOL ABUSE**	**E16**

Go to **E17**, page 58 (*Nonalcohol Substance Use Disorders*).

NONALCOHOL SUBSTANCE USE DISORDERS

Have you ever taken any of these to get high, to sleep better, to lose weight, or to change your mood?

SHOW DRUG LIST (LAST PAGE OF SCORESHEET) TO PATIENT AND RECORD INFORMATION ON SCORESHEET

E17 Which one caused you the most problems?

IF DENIES PROBLEMS: Which one did you use the most?

INDICATE ON SCORESHEET DRUG CLASS WITH HEAVIEST USE/MOST PROBLEMS OR "NONE" IF NO HEAVY DRUG USE AND NO DRUG-RELATED PROBLEMS **E17**

IF Nonalcohol Substance Dependence seems likely, skip to **E23,** page 60.

If "NONE" recorded for **E17,** go to **Module F,** page 65 *(Anxiety and Other Disorders).*

NONALCOHOL SUBSTANCE ABUSE

Now I'd like to ask you some questions about your use of [DRUG USED THE MOST OR CAUSED THE MOST PROBLEMS]. During that time . . .

CRITERIA FOR NONALCOHOL SUBSTANCE ABUSE

A. A maladaptive pattern of substance use leading to clinically significant impairment or distress, as manifested by one (or more) of the following, occurring within a 12-month period:

E18 Did you miss work or school because you were high or very hung over? (How often?) (What about doing a bad job at work or failing courses at school because you used [DRUG]?)

IF NO: What about not keeping your house clean or not taking proper care of your children because of using [DRUG]? (How often?)

(1) recurrent substance use resulting in a failure to fulfill major role obligations at work, school, or home (e.g., repeated absences or poor work performance related to substance use; substance-related absences, suspensions, or expulsions from school; neglect of children or household) **E18**

E19	Did you ever use [DRUG] in a situation in which it might have been dangerous? (Did you ever drive when you were really too high to drive?) IF YES: How often? (When?)	(2) recurrent substance use in situations in which it is physically hazardous (e.g., driving an automobile or operating a machine when impaired by substance use)	**E19**
E20	Did your use of [DRUG] get you into trouble with the law? IF YES: How often? (When?)	(3) recurrent substance-related legal problems (e.g., arrests for substance-related disorderly conduct)	**E20**
E21	IF NOT ALREADY KNOWN: Did your use of [DRUG] cause problems with other people, such as with family members, friends, or people at work? (Did you ever get into physical fights when you were using [DRUG]?) (What about having bad arguments about your drug use?) IF YES: Did you keep on using [DRUG] anyway?	(4) continued substance use despite having persistent or recurrent social or interpersonal problems caused or exacerbated by the effects of the substance (e.g., arguments with spouse about consequences of intoxication, physical fights)	**E21**
E22		**AT LEAST ONE ABUSE ITEM IS "+"**	**E22**

If **E22** is "–" (i.e., no abuse items are "+"), either go back to **E17,** page 58, if the use of any other class of drug may also have been problematic or excessive, or else go to **Module F,** page 65 *(Anxiety and Other Disorders).*

If **E22** is "+" (i.e., at least one abuse item is "+") AND you have already checked for Dependence (i.e., evaluated **E23–E29** on pages 60–61) and found that fewer than 3 were "+," go to **E32,** page 62, and make a diagnosis of *Nonalcohol Substance Abuse.*

NONALCOHOL SUBSTANCE DEPENDENCE

I would now like to ask you some more questions about [TIME WHEN USING THE MOST DRUGS/TIME WHEN DRUGS CAUSED THE MOST PROBLEMS]. During that time . . .

CRITERIA FOR NONALCOHOL SUBSTANCE DEPENDENCE

A maladaptive pattern of substance use, leading to clinically significant impairment or distress, as manifested by three (or more) of the following, occurring at any time in the same 12-month period:

NOTE: Criteria for Dependence are presented in a different order than in DSM-IV.

E23 Did you often find that when you started using [DRUG] you ended up using much more than you were planning to?

IF NO: What about using it for a much longer period of time than you were planning to?

(3) the substance is often taken in larger amounts OR over a longer period than was intended **E23**

E24 Did you try to cut down or stop using [DRUG]?

IF YES: Did you ever actually stop using [DRUG] altogether? (How many times did you try to cut down or stop altogether?)

IF NO: Did you want to stop or cut down? (Is this something you kept worrying about?)

(4) there is a persistent desire OR unsuccessful efforts to cut down or control substance use **E24**

E25 Did you spend a lot of time using [DRUG] or doing whatever you had to do to get it? Did it take you a long time to get back to normal?

(5) a great deal of time is spent in activities necessary to obtain the substance (e.g., visiting multiple doctors or driving long distances), use the substance, or recover from its effects **E25**

E26 Did you have times when you would use [DRUG] so often that you started to use [DRUG] instead of working, spending time with your family or friends, or engaging in other important activities, such as sports, gardening, or playing music?

(6) important social, occupational, or recreational activities are given up or reduced because of substance use **E26**

E27 IF NOT ALREADY KNOWN: Did your drug use cause any psychological problems such as making you depressed or anxious, making it difficult to sleep, or causing "blackouts"?

IF NOT ALREADY KNOWN: Did your drug use cause significant physical problems or make a physical problem worse?

IF YES TO EITHER OF ABOVE: Did you keep on using anyway?

(7) the substance use is continued despite knowledge of having a persistent or recurrent physical or psychological problem that is likely to have been caused or exacerbated by the substance (e.g., current cocaine use despite recognition of cocaine-induced depression) **E27**

E28 Did you find that you needed to use a lot more [DRUG] in order to get the feeling you wanted than you did when you first started using it?

IF YES: How much more?

IF NO: What about finding that when you used the same amount, it had much less effect than before?

(1) tolerance, as defined by either of the following: **E28**

(a) a need for markedly increased amounts of the substance to achieve intoxication or desired effect

(b) markedly diminished effect with continued use of the same amount of the substance

E29 THE FOLLOWING MAY NOT APPLY TO CANNABIS, HALLUCINOGENS, AND PHENCYCLIDINE.

Did you ever have withdrawal symptoms, that is, feel sick when you cut down or stopped using [DRUG]?

IF YES: What symptoms did you have? [REFER TO LIST OF WITHDRAWAL SYMPTOMS ON PAGE 63]

IF HAD WITHDRAWAL SYMPTOMS: After not using [DRUG] for a few hours or more, did you often use it to keep yourself from getting sick with [WITHDRAWAL SYMPTOMS]?

What about using [DRUG IN SAME CLASS] when you were feeling sick with [WITHDRAWAL SYMPTOMS] so that you would feel better?

(2) withdrawal, as manifested by either (a) or (b): **E29**

(a) the characteristic withdrawal syndrome for the substance (see page 61)

(b) the same (or a closely related) substance is taken to relieve or avoid withdrawal symptoms

E30	IF UNKNOWN: When did [SYMPTOMS RATED "+" ABOVE] occur? (Did they all happen around the same time?)	**AT LEAST THREE DEPENDENCE ITEMS (E23–E29) ARE "+" AND OCCURRED WITHIN THE SAME 12-MONTH PERIOD**	E30

If **E30** is "–" (fewer than three dependence items are "+") AND you previously skipped **E18–E21,** pages 58–59 (because dependence seemed likely), return to **E18**, page 58, and check for *Nonalcohol Substance Abuse.*

If **E30** is "–" (fewer than three dependence items are "+") AND **E22,** page 59, is "+" (criteria met for *Nonalcohol Substance Abuse*), go to **E32,** below.

E31	IF UNKNOWN: Have you had [SYMPTOMS RATED "+" ABOVE] in the past month?	**MAKE A DIAGNOSIS OF SUBSTANCE DEPENDENCE**	E31

Go to **Module F**, page 65 *(Anxiety and Other Disorders).*

E32	IF UNKNOWN: Have you had [SYMPTOMS OF ABUSE RATED "+"] in the past month?	**MAKE A DIAGNOSIS OF SUBSTANCE ABUSE**	E32

Go to **Module F**, page 65 *(Anxiety and Other Disorders).*

LIST OF WITHDRAWAL SYMPTOMS (FROM DSM-IV CRITERIA)

Listed below are the characteristic withdrawal symptoms for those classes of substances for which a withdrawal syndrome has been identified. (*NOTE:* A specific withdrawal syndrome has not been identified for CANNABIS and HALLUCINOGENS/PCP.) Withdrawal symptoms may occur following the cessation of prolonged moderate or heavy use of a substance or a reduction in the amount used.

SEDATIVES, HYPNOTICS, AND ANXIOLYTICS: Two (or more) of the following, developing within several hours to a few days after cessation (or reduction) of sedative, hypnotic, or anxiolytic use, that has been heavy and prolonged:

(1) autonomic hyperactivity (e.g., sweating or pulse rate greater than 100)
(2) increased hand tremor
(3) insomnia
(4) nausea or vomiting
(5) transient visual, tactile, or auditory hallucinations or illusions
(6) psychomotor agitation
(7) anxiety
(8) grand mal seizures

STIMULANTS/COCAINE: Dysphoric mood AND two (or more) of the following physiological changes, developing within a few hours to several days after cessation (or reduction of stimulant or cocaine use that has been heavy and prolonged):

(1) fatigue
(2) vivid, unpleasant dreams
(3) insomnia or hypersomnia
(4) increased appetite
(5) psychomotor retardation or agitation

OPIOIDS: Three (or more) of the following, developing within minutes to several days after cessation (or reduction) of opioid use that has been heavy and prolonged (several weeks or longer) or after administration of an opioid antagonist (after a period of opioid use):

(1) dysphoric mood
(2) nausea or vomiting
(3) muscle aches
(4) lacrimation or rhinorrhea
(5) pupillary dilation, piloerection, or sweating
(6) diarrhea
(7) yawning
(8) fever
(9) insomnia

F. ANXIETY AND OTHER DISORDERS

PANIC DISORDER

CRITERIA FOR PANIC DISORDER

F1 Have you ever had a panic attack when you suddenly felt frightened or anxious or suddenly developed a lot of physical symptoms?

IF YES: Have these attacks ever come on completely out of the blue—in situations where you did not expect to be nervous or uncomfortable?

IF UNCLEAR: How many of these kinds of attacks have you had? (At least two?)

A. (1) recurrent unexpected panic attacks **F1**

If **F1** is "–" (i.e., no recurrent unexpected attacks), go to **F25,** page 70 (check for *Obsessive-Compulsive Disorder).*

F2 After any of these attacks...

(2) at least one of the attacks has been followed by 1 month (or more) of one (or more) of the following: **F2**

Did you worry that there might be something terribly wrong with you, like you were having a heart attack or were going crazy? (How long did you worry? At least a month?)

(b) worry about the implications of the attack or its consequences (e.g., losing control, having a heart attack, "going crazy")

IF NO: Did you worry a lot about having another one? (How long did you worry? At least a month?)

(a) persistent concern about having additional attacks

IF NO: Did you do anything differently because of the attacks, like avoiding certain places or not going out alone? (What about avoiding certain activities such as exercise? What about things like always making sure you're near a bathroom or an exit?)

(c) a significant change in behavior related to the attacks

If **F2** is "–" (i.e., no persistent concern about attacks or implications and no change in lifestyle), go to **F25,** page 70 (check for *Obsessive-Compulsive Disorder).*

When was the last bad one? What was the first thing you noticed? Then what?

F3	IF UNKNOWN: Did the symptoms come on all of a sudden? IF YES: How long did it take from when it began to when it got really bad? (Less than 10 minutes?)	The panic attack symptoms developed abruptly and reached a peak within 10 minutes	F3

If **F3** is "–" (i.e., symptoms did not develop abruptly or took longer than 10 minutes to reach peak), go to **F25,** page 70 *(check for Obsessive-Compulsive Disorder).*

During that attack...

F4	... did your heart race, pound, or skip?	(1) palpitations, pounding heart, or accelerated heart rate	F4
F5	... did you sweat?	(2) sweating	F5
F6	... did you tremble or shake?	(3) trembling or shaking	F6
F7	... were you short of breath? (have trouble catching your breath?)	(4) sensations of shortness of breath or smothering	F7
F8	... did you feel as if you were choking?	(5) feeling of choking	F8
F9	... did you have chest pain or pressure?	(6) chest pain or discomfort	F9
F10	... did you have nausea or an upset stomach or the feeling that you were going to have diarrhea?	(7) nausea or abdominal distress	F10
F11	... did you feel dizzy, unsteady, or like you might faint?	(8) feeling dizzy, unsteady, lightheaded, or faint	F11
F12	... did things around you seem unreal or did you feel detached from things around you or detached from parts of your body?	(9) derealization (feelings of unreality) or depersonalization (being detached from oneself)	F12
F13	... were you afraid you were going crazy or might lose control?	(10) fear of losing control or going crazy	F13

F14 . . . were you afraid you might die? — (11) fear of dying **F14**

F15 . . . did you have tingling or numbness in parts of your body? — (12) paresthesias (numbness or tingling sensations) **F15**

F16 . . . did you have flushes (hot flashes) or chills? — (13) chills or hot flushes **F16**

F17 — **AT LEAST FOUR OF F4–F16 ARE "+"** **F17**

> IF **F17** is "–" (i.e., three or fewer symptoms of a panic attack were present), go to **F25,** page 70 (check for *Obsessive-Compulsive Disorder).*

F18 Just before this began, were you physically ill?

Just before this began, were you taking any medications?

IF YES: Any change in the amount you were taking?

Just before this began, were you drinking or using any street drugs?

> If there is any indication that the panic attacks may be secondary (i.e., a direct physiological consequence of a general medical condition or substance), go to page 81 and return here to make rating of "–" or "+."

C. Not due to the direct physiological effects of a substance (e.g., a drug of abuse, medication) or to a general medical condition. **F18**

Etiological general medical conditions include hyperthyroidism, hyperparathyroidism, pheochromocytoma, vestibular dysfunctions, seizure disorders, and cardiac conditions (e.g., arrhythmias, supraventricular tachycardia).

Etiological substances include intoxication with central nervous stimulants (e.g., cocaine, amphetamines, caffeine) or cannabis or withdrawal from central nervous system depressants (e.g., alcohol, barbiturates) or from cocaine.

> If **F18** above is "–" (i.e., panic attacks due to substance or general medical condition), ask the following:
>
> Have there been any other times when you have had panic attacks and they were not because of [GENERAL MEDICAL CONDITION/SUBSTANCE USE]?
>
> If "yes," go back to **F1,** page 65, and ask about those attacks.
> If "no," go to **F25,** page 70 *(check for Obsessive-Compulsive Disorder).*

F19

D. The panic attacks are not better accounted for by another mental disorder, such as Specific Phobia (e.g., on exposure to a specific phobic situation), Obsessive-Compulsive Disorder (e.g., on exposure to dirt in someone with an obsession about contamination), Posttraumatic Stress Disorder (e.g., in response to stimuli associated with a severe stressor), Separation Anxiety Disorder (e.g., in response to being away from home or close relatives), or Social Phobia (e.g., occurring on exposure to feared social situations).

F19

If **F19** is "–" (i.e., panic attacks are better accounted for by another mental disorder), go to **F25,** page 70 *(check for Obsessive-Compulsive Disorder).*

CRITERIA FOR PANIC DISORDER WITH AGORAPHOBIA

F20

IF NOT OBVIOUS FROM OVERVIEW: Are there situations that make you nervous because you are afraid that you might have a panic attack?

IF YES: Tell me about that. . .

IF CANNOT GIVE SPECIFICS: What about. . .

. . . being uncomfortable if you're more than a certain distance from home?
. . . being in a crowded place like a busy store, movie theater, or restaurant?
. . . standing in a line?
. . . being on a bridge?
. . . using public transportation—like a bus, train, or subway—or driving a car?

B. The presence of Agoraphobia:

(1) Anxiety about being in places or situations from which escape might be difficult (or embarrassing) or in which help may not be available in the event of having an unexpected or situationally predisposed panic attack. Agoraphobic fears typically involve characteristic clusters of situations that include being outside the home alone; being in a crowd or standing in a line; being on a bridge; and traveling in a bus, train, or automobile.

F20

If **F20** is "–" (no anxiety about being in places associated with panic attack), go to **F24,** page 69.

F21 Do you avoid these situations?

IF NO: When you are in one of these situations, do you feel very uncomfortable or as if you might have a panic attack?

(Can you go into one of these situations only if you are with someone you know?)

(2) Agoraphobic situations are avoided (e.g., travel is restricted) or else are endured with marked distress or with anxiety about having a panic attack or panic-like symptoms, or require the presence of a companion. **F21**

If **F21** is "–" (i.e., agoraphobic situations are not avoided and there is no distress), go to **F24**, below.

F22

(3) The anxiety or phobic avoidance is not better accounted for by another mental disorder, such as Social Phobia (e.g., avoidance limited to social situations because of fear of embarrassment), Specific Phobia (e.g., avoidance limited to a single situation such as elevators), Obsessive-Compulsive Disorder (e.g., avoidance of dirt in someone with an obsession about contamination), Posttraumatic Stress Disorder (e.g., avoidance of stimuli associated with a severe stressor), or Separation Anxiety Disorder (e.g., avoidance of leaving home or relatives). **F22**

If **F22** is "–" (i.e., avoidance is better accounted for by another mental disorder), go to **F24**, below.

F23 IF UNKNOWN: Have you had [PANIC ATTACKS OR SYMPTOMS OF AGORAPHOBIA] in the past month?

AGORAPHOBIA IS PRESENT WITH PANIC DISORDER. (MAKE A DIAGNOSIS OF 300.21 PANIC DISORDER WITH AGORAPHOBIA) **F23**

Go to **F25**, page 70 (check for *Obsessive-Compulsive Disorder*).

F24 IF UNKNOWN: Have you had any panic attacks in the past month?

AGORAPHOBIA IS <u>NOT</u> PRESENT WITH PANIC DISORDER. (MAKE A DIAGNOSIS OF 300.01 PANIC DISORDER WITHOUT AGORAPHOBIA) **F24**

Go to **F25**, page 70 (check for *Obsessive-Compulsive Disorder*).

OBSESSIVE-COMPULSIVE DISORDER

CRITERIA FOR OBSESSIVE-COMPULSIVE DISORDER

F25 Now I would like to ask you if you have ever been bothered by thoughts that did not make any sense and kept coming back to you even when you tried not to have them?

(What were they?)

IF PATIENT NOT SURE WHAT IS MEANT: . . . Thoughts like hurting someone even though you really did not want to, or being contaminated by germs or dirt?

Obsessions are defined by (1), (2), (3), and (4):

(1) recurrent and persistent thoughts, impulses, or images that are experienced, at some time during the disturbance, as intrusive and inappropriate and that cause marked anxiety or distress **F25**

> If **F25** is "–" (i.e., no recurrent thoughts that are intrusive and inappropriate), go to **F30**, page 71.

F26

(2) the thoughts, impulses, or images are not simply excessive worries about real-life problems **F26**

> If **F26** is "–" (i.e., thoughts are simply worries about real-life problems), go to **F30,** page 71.

F27 When you had these thoughts, did you try hard to get them out of your head? (What would you try to do?)

(3) the person attempts to ignore or suppress such thoughts, impulses, or images or to neutralize them with some other thought or action **F27**

> If **F27** is "–" (i.e., no attempt to ignore or suppress thoughts), go to **F30**, page 71.

F28 IF UNCLEAR: Where do you think these thoughts are coming from?

(4) the person recognizes that the obsessional thoughts, impulses, or images are a product of his or her own mind (not imposed from without as in thought insertion) **F28**

> If **F28** is "–" (i.e., person feels thoughts are imposed from without), go to **F30,** page 71.

F29

OBSESSIONS (1), (2), (3), AND (4) ARE "+" **F29**

F30	Was there ever anything that you had to do over and over again and could not resist doing, such as washing your hands again and again, counting up to a certain number, or checking something several times to make sure you had done it right? (What did you have to do?)	Compulsions as defined by (1) and (2): (1) repetitive behaviors (e.g., hand washing, ordering, checking) or mental acts (praying, counting, repeating words silently) that the person feels driven to perform in response to an obsession, or according to certain rules that must be applied rigidly	**F30**

> If **F30** is "–" (i.e., no repetitive behaviors or mental acts in response to obsession or according to rules), go to **F33**, below.

F31	IF UNCLEAR: Why did you have to do [COMPULSIVE ACT]? What would happen if you did not do it? IF UNCLEAR: How many times would you do [COMPULSIVE ACT]? How much time a day would you spend doing it?	(2) the behaviors or mental acts are aimed at preventing or reducing distress or preventing some dreaded event or situation; however, these behaviors or mental acts either are not connected in a realistic way with what they are designed to prevent or neutralize or are clearly excessive	**F31**

> If **F31** is "–" (i.e., behaviors or acts are not aimed at preventing distress or some dreaded event and are not excessive), go to **F33**, below.

F32		**COMPULSIONS (1) AND (2) ARE "+"**	**F32**
F33	**EITHER F29 IS "+" OR F32 IS "+"**	A. Either obsessions or compulsions	**F33**

> If **F33** is "–" (i.e., neither obsessions nor compulsions present), go to **F39**, page 73 *(check for Posttraumatic Stress Disorder).*

F34	Have you (thought about [OBSESSIVE THOUGHTS]/done [COMPULSIVE ACTS]) more than you should have (or than made sense)? IF NO: How about when you first started having this problem?	B. At some point during the course of the disorder, the person has recognized that the obsessions or compulsions are excessive or unreasonable. **Note:** This does not apply to children.	**F34**

> If **F34** is "–" (i.e., never recognized that obsessions or compulsions are unreasonable), go to **F39**, page 73 *(check for Posttraumatic Stress Disorder).*

F35 What effect does this [OBSESSION OR COMPULSION] have on your life? (Did [OBSESSION OR COMPULSION] bother you a lot? How much time have you spent on [OBSESSION OR COMPULSION]?)

C. The obsessions or compulsions cause marked distress, are time-consuming (take more than an hour a day), or significantly interfere with the person's normal routine, occupational functioning, or usual social activities or relationships. **F35**

If **F35** is "–" (i.e., obsessions and compulsions not clinically significant), go to **F39**, page 73 *(check for Posttraumatic Stress Disorder).*

F36

D. If another Axis I disorder is present, the content of the obsessions or compulsions is not restricted to it (e.g., preoccupation with food in the presence of an Eating Disorder; hair pulling in the presence of Trichotillomania; concern with appearance in the presence of Body Dysmorphic Disorder; preoccupation with drugs in the presence of a Substance Use Disorder; preoccupation with having a serious illness in the presence of Hypochondriasis; preoccupation with sexual urges or fantasies in the presence of a Paraphilia; or guilty ruminations in the presence of Major Depressive Disorder). **F36**

If **F36** is "–" (i.e., the content of obsessions and compulsions is restricted to another Axis I disorder), go to **F39**, page 73 *(check for Posttraumatic Stress Disorder).*

F37 Just before you began having [OBSESSIONS OR COMPULSIONS] were you taking any drugs or medicines?

Just before the [OBSESSIONS OR COMPULSIONS] started, were you physically ill?

If there is any indication that the obsessions or compulsions may be secondary (i.e., a direct physiological consequence of a general medical condition or substance), go to page 81 and return here to make rating of "–" or "+."

E. Not due to the direct physiological effects of a substance (e.g., a drug of abuse, a medication) or a general medical condition. **F37**

Etiological general medical conditions include certain central nervous system neoplasms.

Etiological substances include intoxication with central nervous system stimulants (e.g., cocaine, amphetamines).

If **F37** is "–" (i.e., the obsessions and compulsions are due to general medical condition or substance), go to **F39**, page 73 *(check for Posttraumatic Stress Disorder).*

F38 IF UNKNOWN: Have you had [OBSESSIONS OR COMPULSIONS] in the past month?

CRITERIA A, B, C, D, AND E ARE "+" (MAKE A DIAGNOSIS OF 300.3 OBSESSIVE-COMPULSIVE DISORDER) **F38**

POSTTRAUMATIC STRESS DISORDER

F39 Sometimes things happen to people that are extremely upsetting—things such as being in a life-threatening situation such as a major disaster, very serious accident or fire; being physically assaulted or raped; seeing another person killed or dead, or badly hurt, or hearing about something horrible that has happened to someone you are close to. At any time during your life, have any of these kinds of things happened to you?

IF ANY EVENTS LISTED: Sometimes these things keep coming back in nightmares, flashbacks, or thoughts that you can't get rid of. Has that ever happened to you?

IF NO: What about being very upset when you were in a situation that reminded you of one of these terrible things?

RECORD TRAUMATIC EVENTS ON SCORESHEET. **F39**

If no events listed or answer to both of above questions is no, go to **F65**, page 77.

FOR FOLLOWING QUESTIONS, FOCUS ON TRAUMATIC EVENT(S) MENTIONED IN SCREENING QUESTION ABOVE.

CRITERIA FOR PTSD

A. The person has been exposed to a traumatic event in which both of the following were present:

F40 IF MORE THAN ONE TRAUMA IS REPORTED: Which of these do you think affected you the most?

(1) the person experienced, witnessed, or was confronted with an event or events that involved actual or threatened death or serious injury, or a threat to the physical integrity of self or others **F40**

If **F40** is "–" (i.e., no qualifying stressor), go to **F65**, page 77.

F41 IF UNCLEAR: How did you react when [TRAUMA] happened? (Were you very afraid or did you feel terrified or helpless?)

(2) the person's response involved intense fear, helplessness, or horror. **F41**

Note: In children, this may be expressed instead by disorganized or agitated behavior.

If **F41** is "–" (i.e., person did not react with fear, helplessness, or horror), go to **F65**, page 77.

Now I would like to ask a few questions about specific ways that it may have affected you.

For example...

B. The traumatic event is persistently reexperienced in one (or more) of the the following ways:

F42 ... did you think about [TRAUMA] when you did not want to or did thoughts about [TRAUMA] come to you suddenly when you didn't want them to?

(1) recurrent and intrusive distressing recollections of the event, including images, thoughts, or perceptions **F42**

Note: In young children, repetitive play may occur in which themes or aspects of the trauma are expressed.

F43 ... what about having dreams about [TRAUMA]?

(2) recurrent distressing dreams of the event **F43**

Note: In children, there may be frightening dreams without recognizable content.

F44 ... what about finding yourself acting or feeling as if you were back in the situation?

(3) acting or feeling as if the traumatic event were recurring (includes a sense of reliving the experience, illusions, hallucinations, and dissociative flashback episodes, including those that occur on awakening or when intoxicated) **F44**

F45 ... what about getting very upset when something reminded you of [TRAUMA]?

(4) intense psychological distress at exposure to internal or external cues that symbolize or resemble an aspect of the traumatic event **F45**

Note: In young children, trauma-specific reenactment may occur.

F46 ... what about having physical symptoms—such as breaking out in a sweat, breathing heavily or irregularly, or your heart pounding or racing?

(5) physiological reactivity on exposure to internal or external cues that symbolize or resemble an aspect of the traumatic event **F46**

F47

AT LEAST ONE "B" SYMPTOM IS "+" **F47**

If **F47** is "–" (i.e., no "B" symptoms are "+"), go to **F65**, page 77.

C. Persistent avoidance of stimuli associated with the trauma and numbing of general responsiveness (not present before the trauma), as indicated by three (or more) of the following:

Since [TRAUMA]...

F48	... have you made a special effort to avoid thinking or talking about what happened?	(1) efforts to avoid thoughts, feelings, or conversations associated with the trauma	**F48**
F49	... have you stayed away from things or people that reminded you of [TRAUMA]?	(2) efforts to avoid activities, places, or people that arouse recollections of the trauma	**F49**
F50	... have you been unable to remember some important part of what happened?	(3) inability to recall an important aspect of the trauma	**F50**
F51	... have you been much less interested in doing things that used to be important to you, such as seeing friends, reading books, or watching TV?	(4) markedly diminished interest or participation in significant activities	**F51**
F52	... have you felt distant or cut off from others?	(5) feeling of detachment or estrangement from others	**F52**
F53	... have you felt "numb" or as if you no longer had strong feelings about anything or loving feelings for anyone?	(6) restricted range of affect (e.g., unable to have loving feelings)	**F53**
F54	... did you notice a change in the way you think about or plan for the future?	(7) sense of a foreshortened future (e.g., does not expect to have a career, marriage, children, or a normal life span)	**F54**
F55		**AT LEAST 3 "C" SYMPTOMS ARE "+"**	**F55**

If **F55** is "–" (i.e., fewer than three "C" symptoms are "+"), go to **F65**, page 77.

D. Persistent symptoms of increased arousal (not present before the trauma), as indicated by two (or more) of the following:

Since [TRAUMA]. . .

F56	. . . have you had trouble sleeping? (What kind of trouble?)	(1) difficulty falling or staying asleep	F56
F57	. . . have you been unusually irritable? What about outbursts of anger?	(2) irritability or outbursts of anger	F57
F58	. . . have you had trouble concentrating?	(3) difficulty concentrating	F58
F59	. . . have you been watchful or on guard even when there was no reason to be?	(4) hypervigilance	F59
F60	. . . have you been jumpy or easily startled, such as by sudden noises?	(5) exaggerated startle response	F60
F61		**AT LEAST TWO "D" SYMPTOMS ARE "+"**	F61

If **F61** is "–" (i.e., fewer than two "D" symptoms are "+"), go to **F65**, page 77.

F62	About how long did these problems, such as [PTSD SYMPTOMS], last?	E. Duration of the disturbance (symptoms in criteria B, C, and D) is more than 1 month.	F62

If **F62** is "–" (i.e., duration is 1 month or less), go to **F65**, page 77.

F63		F. The disturbance causes clinically significant distress or impairment in social, occupational, or other important areas of functioning.	F63

If **F63** is "–" (i.e., disturbance is not clinically significant), go to **F65**, page 77.

F64	IF UNKNOWN: Have you had [SYMPTOMS CODED "+"] in the past month?	**CRITERIA A, B, C, D, E, AND F ARE "+"** (MAKE A DIAGNOSIS OF 309.81 POSTTRAUMATIC STRESS DISORDER)	F64

OTHER ANXIETY DISORDERS

F65 IF PANIC DISORDER NOT ALREADY DIAGNOSED: Were you ever afraid of going out of the house alone, being alone, being in a crowd, standing in a line, or traveling on buses or trains?

IF YES, Consider: **300.22 Agoraphobia Without History of Panic Disorder** (DSM-IV pages 404–405). Agoraphobia related to the fear of developing panic-like symptoms (e.g., dizziness or diarrhea) without a history of Panic Disorder **F65**

F66 Is there anything that you have been afraid to do or felt uncomfortable doing in front of other people, such as speaking, eating, or writing?

IF YES, Consider: **300.23 Social Phobia** (DSM-IV pages 416–417). Marked and persistent fear of one or more social (or performance) situations that interferes significantly with the person's normal routine, occupational functioning, social activities or relationships (or there is marked distress about having the phobia) **F66**

F67 Are there any other things that you have been especially afraid of, such as flying, seeing blood, getting a shot, heights, closed places, or certain kinds of animals or insects?

IF YES, Consider: **300.29 Specific Phobia** (DSM-IV pages 410–411). Marked and persistent fear that is excessive and unreasonable that interferes significantly with the person's normal routine, occupational functioning, social activities, or relationships (or there is marked distress about having the phobia) **F67**

F68 In the past 6 months, have you been particularly nervous or anxious?

IF YES, Consider: **300.02 Generalized Anxiety Disorder** (DSM-IV pages 435–436). Excessive anxiety and worry more days than not for at least 6 months, not due to a general medical condition or substance, causing significant distress or impairment.
NOTE: A diagnosis of Generalized Anxiety Disorder requires that the anxiety occur at times other than exclusively during a Mood or Psychotic Disorder. **F68**

ANXIETY DISORDER NOT OTHERWISE SPECIFIED

F69

Clinically significant anxiety or phobic avoidance that does not meet criteria for any specific Anxiety Disorder, Adjustment Disorder With Anxiety, or Adjustment Disorder With Mixed Anxiety and Depressed Mood **F69**

If **F69** is "–" (i.e., absence of clinically significant anxiety symptoms not meeting criteria for a specific Anxiety Disorder), go to **F72**, page 78 *(Somatoform Disorders).*

F70 Just before this began, were you physically ill?

Just before this began, were you taking any medications?

IF YES: Any change in the amount you were taking?

Just before this began, were you drinking or taking any street drugs?

If there is any indication that the anxiety symptoms may be secondary (i.e., a direct physiological consequence of a general medical condition or substance), go to page 81 and return here to make rating of "–" or "+."

Not due to the direct physiological effects of a substance (e.g., a drug of abuse, medication) or to a general medical condition **F70**

Etiological general medical conditions include hyper- and hypothyroidism, hypoglycemia, hyperparathyroidism, pheochromocytoma, congestive heart failure, arrhythmias, pulmonary embolism, chronic obstructive pulmonary disease, pneumonia, hyperventilation, vitamin B_{12} deficiency, porphyria, central nervous system neoplasms, vestibular dysfunction, and encephalitis.

Etiological substances include intoxication with central nervous system stimulants (e.g., cocaine, amphetamines, caffeine) or cannabis, hallucinogens, PCP, or alcohol, or withdrawal from central nervous system depressants (e.g., alcohol, sedatives, hypnotics).

If **F70** is "–" (i.e., due to a substance or general medical condition), go to **F72,** below.

F71 IF UNKNOWN: Have you had [ANXIETY SYMPTOMS] in the past month?

MAKE A DIAGNOSIS OF 300.00 ANXIETY DISORDER NOT OTHERWISE SPECIFIED **F71**

SOMATOFORM DISORDERS

F72 Over the past several years, what has your physical health been like?

How often have you had to go to a doctor because you weren't feeling well? (What for?)

IF OFTEN: Was the doctor always able to find out what was wrong? (Tell me about that.) Were there times when the doctor said there was nothing wrong but you were still convinced that something was wrong?)

If there have been unexplained physical complaints, consider: **F72**

300.81 Somatization Disorder (DSM-IV pages 449–450). At least eight unexplained physical complaints occurring over a period of several years, beginning before age 30 ***OR***

300.82 Undifferentiated Somatoform Disorder (DSM-IV pages 451–452). Unexplained physical complaints that do not meet criteria for Somatization Disorder

F73 Do you worry much about your physical health? Does your doctor think you worry too much?

IF YES, Consider: **300.7 Hypochondriasis** (DSM-IV page 465). Preoccupation with fears of having a serious illness that persist despite appropriate medical evaluation and assurance **F73**

F74 Some people are very bothered by the way they look. Is this a problem for you?

IF YES, Consider: **300.7 Body Dysmorphic Disorder** (DSM-IV page 468). Preoccupation with an imagined defect in appearance **F74**

EATING DISORDERS

F75 Have you ever had a time when you weighed much less than other people thought you ought to weigh?

IF YES, Consider: **307.1 Anorexia Nervosa** (DSM-IV pages 544–545). Refusal to maintain body weight at or above a minimally normal weight, accompanied by an intense fear of becoming fat **F75**

F76 Have you often had times when your eating was out of control?

Tell me about those times.

IF YES, Consider: **307.51 Bulimia Nervosa** (DSM-IV pages 549–550). Recurrent episodes of binge eating with inappropriate compensatory behavior **F76**

CONTINUE WITH THE REMAINDER OF THE SCID ONLY IF THERE IS A CURRENT DISTURBANCE AND IT DOES NOT MEET THE CRITERIA FOR A SPECIFIC AXIS I DSM-IV DISORDER, OTHERWISE **END SCID.**

ADJUSTMENT DISORDERS

CRITERIA FOR ADJUSTMENT DISORDERS

F77 IF UNKNOWN: Did anything happen to you just before [ONSET OF CURRENT DISTURBANCE]?

IF YES: Do you think that [STRESSOR] had anything to do with your getting [SYMPTOMS]?

A. The development of emotional or behavioral symptoms in response to an identifiable stressor(s) occurring within 3 months of the onset of the stressor(s) **F77**

If **F77** is "–" (i.e., no symptoms in response to a stressor), **END SCID.**

F78 (What effect have [SYMPTOMS] had on you and your ability to do things? How upset were you? Has it made it hard for you to do your work or be with friends?)

B. These symptoms or behaviors are clinically significant as evidenced by either of the following:

(1) marked distress that is in excess of what would be expected from exposure to the stressor

(2) significant impairment in social or occupational (academic) functioning. **F78**

If **F78** is "–" (i.e., symptoms not clinically significant), **END SCID.**

F79 (Have you had this kind of reaction many times before?)

(Were you having [SYMPTOMS] even before [STRESSOR] happened?)

C. The stress-related disturbance does not meet the criteria for another specific Axis I disorder and is not merely an exacerbation of a preexisting Axis I or Axis II disorder. **F79**

If **F79** is "–" (i.e., exacerbation of preexisting disorder), **END SCID.**

F80 IF UNKNOWN: Did someone close to you die just before [ONSET OF CURRENT DISTURBANCE]?

D. The symptoms do not represent Bereavement. **F80**

If **F80** is "–" (i.e., represents Bereavement), **END SCID.**

F81 (How long has it been now since [STRESSOR AND COMPLICATIONS ARISING FROM STRESSOR] were over?)

E. Once the stressor (or its consequences) has terminated, the symptoms do not persist for more than an additional 6 months. **F81**

If **F81** is "–" (i.e., symptoms persisted 6 months beyond termination of stressor), make the appropriate Not Otherwise Specified diagnosis (i.e., go to **D17**, page 52, if depressive symptoms or **F69**, page 77, if anxiety symptoms).

F82 **Make diagnosis of Adjustment Disorder based on predominant symptoms:** **F82**

309.0 Adjustment Disorder With Depressed Mood
309.24 Adjustment Disorder With Anxiety
309.28 Adjustment Disorder With Mixed Anxiety and Depressed Mood
309.3 Adjustment Disorder With Disturbance of Conduct
309.4 Adjustment Disorder With Mixed Disturbance of Emotions and Conduct
309.9 Unspecified Adjustment Disorder

END SCID

CONSIDER ETIOLOGICAL ROLE OF A GENERAL MEDICAL CONDITION OR SUBSTANCE USE

If panic attacks, obsessions, compulsions, or other anxiety symptoms are not temporally associated with a general medical condition, go to **F87**, page 83 (*Substance-Induced Anxiety Disorder*).

ANXIETY DISORDER DUE TO A GENERAL MEDICAL CONDITION

F83 CODE BASED ON INFORMATION ALREADY OBTAINED

F84 Do you think your [PANIC ATTACKS/ OBSESSIONS/COMPULSIONS/ANXIETY SYMPTOMS] were in any way related to your [COMORBID GENERAL MEDICAL CONDITION]?

IF YES: Tell me how.

(Did the [PANIC ATTACKS/OBSESSIONS/COMPULSIONS/ANXIETY SYMPTOMS] start or get much worse only after [COMORBID GENERAL MEDICAL CONDITION] began?)

IF YES AND GENERAL MEDICAL CONDITION HAS RESOLVED: Did the [PANIC ATTACKS/ OBSESSIONS/COMPULSIONS/ ANXIETY SYMPTOMS] get better once the [COMORBID GENERAL MEDICAL CONDITION] got better?

CRITERIA FOR ANXIETY DISORDER DUE TO A GENERAL MEDICAL CONDITION

A. Prominent anxiety, panic attacks, or obsessions or compulsions predominate in the clinical picture. **F83**

B/C. There is evidence from the history, physical examination, or laboratory findings that the disturbance is the direct physiological consequence of a general medical condition, and the disturbance is not better accounted for by another mental disorder (e.g., Adjustment Disorder With Anxiety in which the stressor is a serious general medical condition). **F84**

If **F84** is "–" (general medical condition not etiological), go to **F87**, page 83 (*Substance-Induced Anxiety Disorder*).

F85	IF UNCLEAR: How much did [PANIC ATTACKS/OBSESSIONS/COMPULSIONS/ ANXIETY SYMPTOMS] interfere with your life?	E. The symptoms cause clinically significant distress or impairment in social, occupational, or other important areas of functioning.	F85
F86	IF UNKNOWN: Have you had [ANXIETY SYMPTOMS] in the past month?	**CRITERIA A, B/C, AND E ARE "+"** (MAKE A DIAGNOSIS OF 293.84 ANXIETY DISORDER DUE TO A GENERAL MEDICAL CONDITION)	F86

If panic attacks, obsessions, compulsions, or other anxiety symptoms are not temporally associated with substance use, return to disorder being evaluated:

F18 for Panic Disorder (page 67)

F37 for Obsessive-Compulsive Disorder (page 72)

F70 for Anxiety Disorder Not Otherwise Specified (page 78)

SUBSTANCE-INDUCED ANXIETY DISORDER

CRITERIA FOR SUBSTANCE-INDUCED ANXIETY DISORDER

F87 CODE BASED ON INFORMATION ALREADY OBTAINED

A. Prominent anxiety, panic attacks, or obsessions or compulsions predominate in the clinical picture. **F87**

F88 IF NOT KNOWN: When did the [PANIC ATTACKS/OBSESSIONS/COMPULSIONS/ ANXIETY SYMPTOMS] begin? Were you already using [SUBSTANCE] or had you just stopped or cut down your use?

B. There is evidence from the history, physical examination, or laboratory findings that either (1) the symptoms in criterion A developed during or within a month of Substance Intoxication or Withdrawal or (2) medication use is etiologically related to the disturbance. **F88**

If **F88** is "–" (i.e., not etiologically related to a substance), return to disorder being evaluated:
F18 for Panic Disorder (page 67)
F37 for Obsessive-Compulsive Disorder (page 72)
F70 for Anxiety Disorder Not Otherwise Specified (page 78)

F89 Do you think your [PANIC ATTACKS/ OBSESSIONS/COMPULSIONS/ ANXIETY SYMPTOMS] are in any way related to your [SUBSTANCE USE]?

IF YES: Tell me how.

ASK ANY OF THE FOLLOWING QUESTIONS AS NEEDED TO RULE OUT NONSUBSTANCE ETIOLOGY

C. The disturbance is not better accounted for by an Anxiety Disorder that is not substance induced. Evidence that the symptoms are better accounted for by an Anxiety Disorder that is not substance induced might include: **F89**

IF UNKNOWN: Which came first, the [SUBSTANCE USE] or the [PANIC ATTACKS/OBSESSIONS/ COMPULSIONS/ANXIETY SYMPTOMS]?

(1) the anxiety symptoms precede the onset of the substance use (or medication use)

IF UNKNOWN: Have you had a period of time when you stopped using [SUBSTANCE]?

IF YES: After you stopped using [SUBSTANCE] did the [PANIC ATTACKS/ANXIETY SYMPTOMS] get better?

(2) the anxiety symptoms persist for a substantial period of time (e.g., about a month) after the cessation of acute withdrawal or severe intoxication

F89 (cont'd)

IF UNKNOWN: How much of [SUBSTANCE] were you using when you began to have [PANIC ATTACKS/ OBSESSIONS/ COMPULSIONS/ANXIETY SYMPTOMS]?

IF UNKNOWN: Have you had any other episodes of [PANIC ATTACKS/ OBSESSIONS/ COMPULSIONS/ANXIETY SYMPTOMS]?

IF YES: How many? Were you using [SUBSTANCE] at those times?

(3) the anxiety symptoms are substantially in excess of what would be expected given the type or amount of the substance used or the duration of use

(4) there is other evidence suggesting the existence of an independent non-substance-induced Anxiety Disorder (e.g., a history of recurrent non-substance-related panic attacks)

F89 (cont'd)

If **F89** is "–" (i.e., the disturbance is better accounted for by a non-substance-induced Anxiety Disorder), return to disorder being evaluated:
F18 for Panic Disorder (page 67)
F37 for Obsessive-Compulsive Disorder (page 72)
F70 for Anxiety Disorder Not Otherwise Specified (page 78)

F90

IF UNKNOWN: How much did [PANIC ATTACKS/OBSESSIONS/COMPULSIONS/ ANXIETY SYMPTOMS] interfere with your life?

E. The symptoms cause clinically significant distress or impairment in social, occupational, or other important areas of functioning.

F90

If **F90** is "–" (not clinically significant), return to disorder being evaluated:
F18 for Panic Disorder (page 67)
F37 for Obsessive-Compulsive Disorder (page 72)
F70 for Anxiety Disorder Not Otherwise Specified (page 78)

F91

IF UNKNOWN: Have you had [ANXIETY SYMPTOMS] in the past month?

CRITERIA A, B, C, AND E ARE "+"
(MAKE A DIAGNOSIS OF SUBSTANCE-INDUCED ANXIETY DISORDER)

F91

Return to disorder being evaluated:
F18 for Panic Disorder (page 67)
F37 for Obsessive-Compulsive Disorder (page 72)
F70 for Anxiety Disorder Not Otherwise Specified (page 78)